LETTERS OF LOVE

TO OUR NEW BREAST FRIENDS

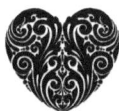

SO BRAVE

SO BRAVE

So Brave is Australia's only Young Women's Breast Cancer Charity, highlighting the unmet needs of Australia's young women.

OUR MISSION

1. EMPOWER young women diagnosed with breast cancer;
2. raise AWARENESS in young women to be #breastaware;
3. EDUCATE young women;
4. fundraise for breast cancer RESEARCH, and;
5. create a LEGACY that changes the conversation.

Our multi-award winning, nationally recognised charity is known for 'punching well above our weight' – we may be small, but our size is our superpower.

OUR VISION

Changing the conversation about young women and breast cancer in Australia through increased awareness of breast cancer in young women, early diagnosis and best survival outcomes.

From the outset, So Brave has been bringing young breast cancer survivors together to share their stories, be empowered through unique artistic experiences and inspire others. We have grown to deliver targetted education workshops at schools, in conjunction with university students and at community events across Australia.

If you would like to support young women in receiving this book, or would like to learn more about our support, programs and ways to get involved, please contact us today.

978-0-6487992-3-8

Please keep following our journey:

f 🐦 ◎ /SOBRAVEOFFICIAL

#SOBRAVE #SOBRAVEOFFICIAL #FEELITONTHEFIFTH #YOUNGBREASTCANCER #BREASTCANCERAWARENESS

SOBRAVE.ORG.AU

CONNECTING THROUGH LETTERS OF LOVE

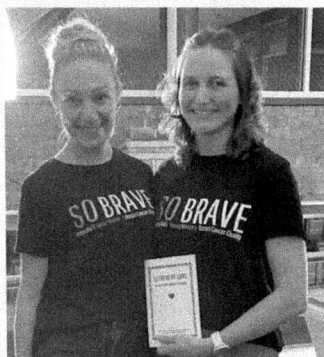

We are two young Aussie breast cancer warriors, Rachel and Claire from Tassie, who connected through this book. We have both walked this journey in our early 30s and with a young family; we have both felt the terror, the overwhelm and the isolation that you are probably feeling right now. We have also been blessed to find connection – that rainbow of hope and empathy that helps to brighten the darkness. The power of connection cannot be underestimated. There is an inexplicable feeling of being understood and validated by talking with others who share your experiences. Being young with breast cancer can be a very lonely place.

RACHEL

In 2020 I was asked to meet with the beautiful Claire, who had just been diagnosed with breast cancer. She was surrounded with incredible supporters, but being so young with three little kiddies, Claire felt so incredibly alone. A feeling I knew all too well. I remember Claire looking at me through tears asking if I feared for my own daughters. If that fear subsides. Neither of our families had a history of breast cancer, but just like that – they suddenly did. I looked back at Claire, also fighting tears, and we looked down at our girls happily playing away. This is why awareness matters. This is what we research for. The next generation.

Breast cancer does happen to women in their 20s and 30s. Unfortunately the younger you are, the more aggressive it usually is. The chances of it sneaking back up on you are high. Too high.

When I met up with Claire I gave her this little book I had stumbled across and wished I had read at the start of my own personal dance with the devil. Written by young fighters from the 'So Brave' community – I read it and no longer felt so isolated. I was filled with hope. Claire read it and felt the same. She's taken a step further and has decided to be a 'So Brave' ambassador for Tasmania. She's also an incredibly brave breast cancer survivor. So Brave's Ambassadors spread awareness to and for young women, that this disease can and does happen to young women also. But - if it does, you're not alone.

1

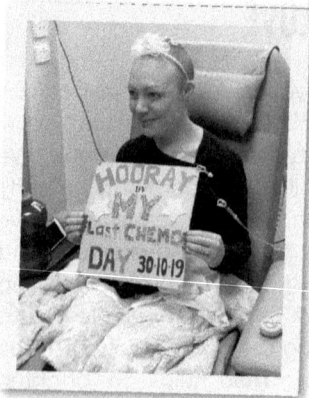

Be Brave like the women you'll read about in this book. Be self aware. If you're 40+ you are eligible for a free mammogram annually. If you're younger – it's all on you to self check each month and act immediately.

Thank you also to my Mum and Dad for buying a bundle of these books and donating them to the breast care nurses in Hobart, to give to any other terrified young women in those early daunting and isolating days.

Claire and I have both learned the fear never does subside. But, you grow stronger and braver. And you cope. You find yourself having more brighter days than dark days. You educate yourself and others, when you feel strong and brave enough to do so. I was diagnosed in 2019 and have undergone lumpectomy surgery, chemotherapy, radiation and lymphoedema treatment. I have also undergone an oophorectomy and take ongoing hormone blockers which is no picnic, especially at such a young age. Like all of us when we are told not to, I found myself Googling - anything and everything – searching for an experience like mine to connect to. Just like Alice, we follow the rabbit down the hole, but cancer it is no Wonderland. On one of my Googling rampages, my search of 'Breast Cancer + Young Women' led me to So Brave. I ordered the book, 'Letters of Love' and after reading it, I found myself feeling less alone.

I didn't personally know these beautiful, brave young women, but here they were, reassuring me, validating me and connecting with me. I only wish I had stumbled on this book earlier in my journey. When the opportunity arose to connect with Claire in 2020 and offer support, I wanted to share this book and the connection it offered.

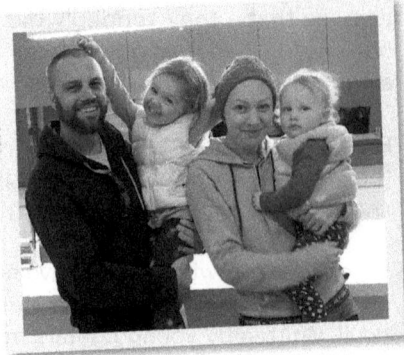

CLAIRE

I was diagnosed in April 2020 just as the world was shutting down due to the pandemic. Being young with breast cancer is uncommon and isolating at any time, but with all the support groups and services closing down at the exact time I was reaching out, I felt so alone,

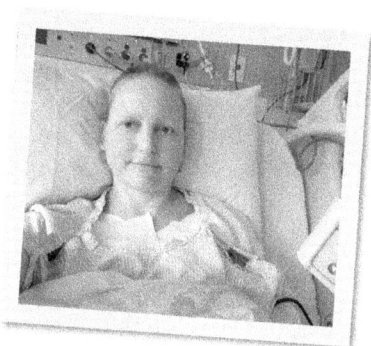

despite my amazing family wrapping me in love and comfort. My treatment included neoadjuvant chemo, bilateral mastectomy and reconstructive surgery (still ongoing) as well as being treated for red-breast syndrome and cording. I was put in touch with Rachel through a mutual contact, and when people were allowed to have a visitor in their home again, we met at my house for a cuppa. Here was another young woman about 18 months ahead of me on this same journey, offering support, answering my millions of questions and selflessly sharing her experience. The connection we both felt was empowering. We chatted for a long time. We both had young families and we connected over the shared fears, hope and uncertainties that come with being a young parent with cancer - have I passed on a genetic fault to my children? Will I still be alive to mother my children? If my daughters do develop breast cancer, will I still be here to support them in the way my mother has supported me? Will we be OK?

Neither of our families had a history of breast cancer, and just like that, suddenly they did. We looked at each other through tears, Claire asked Rachel if she worried about her daughters? Does that fear subside? We both looked at our girls, playing innocently together nearby and Rachel answered that the fear does not subside, but you learn to live with it - you learn to be braver than your fear, stronger than your pain. This is why we research, for the next generation, and this is why we connect - to give each other the strength to be braver than our fears. We connected over the stories of these other young women who had shared their stories - the letters in this book from beautiful, brave, empowering young women.

These women gave Rachel hope and strength. And in turn, Rachel gave me hope and strength, and together we urge you to connect in - you are not alone in this crappy hand you have been dealt. You are stronger than you realise. We are OK - and you will be too. You have found So Brave, and darling, we know you are scared and we are here for you.

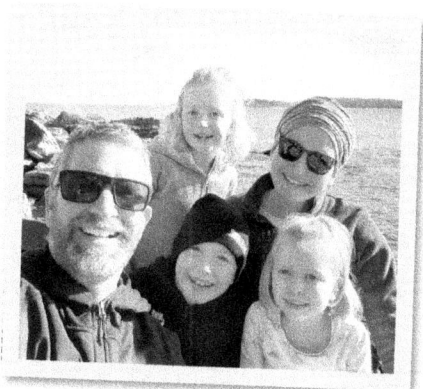

We were both incredibly lucky to have a wonderful army of supporters behind us on our respective journeys – and that is something to be grateful for. Our supporters are incredible and provide us so much strength, but when we found the connection of someone else in our shoes – another breast cancer warrior walking in the trenches with us, totally understanding and pre-empting the ways in which we will fall and offering us a hand back up and advice on where to step next, that is when we no longer felt quite so terrified. You are not alone.

We are both passionate about getting awareness out into our communities and paying forward support to you and other young women that follow after us. Rachel and her family have continued to offer support by passing this very book on to local cancer clinics to give to young breast cancer patients - people like you maybe. Claire has taken on a So Brave ambassadorship in 2022 to raise awareness and funds for research, education and supports for our next generation of young women. We are humbled to be able to share our connection with you in this book that holds very special meaning to both of us. We have experienced the empowering connection from reading these letters of love. We hope, as you read this book, you too will find hope, validation, some insights into what may be coming up for you and most of all connection, because, beautiful and brave one – you are not alone.

♡ *Rachel & Claire*

PAY IT FORWARD

Please donate to So Brave today or get in touch to arrange a bulk buy to donate to your local cancer centre or specialist's office.

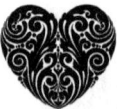

VISIT: SOBRAVE.ORG.AU/DONATE/
CALL: 07 3103 2377
EMAIL: TEAM@SOBRAVE.COM.AU

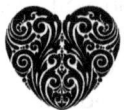

FOREWORD

I first became aware of So Brave in 2017, soon after my Aunty Judy went through treatment for breast cancer, and not long after my brother Dave passed away from oesophageal cancer. Dave was diagnosed on 5th August 2016 and passed away on the 29th August 2016 with his partner and four children by his side, and a room full of his loved ones. Just three short weeks after diagnosis...

Looking back, those three weeks were beyond overwhelming. As someone without a medical background, keeping up with the doctor's reports was confusing and difficult. Desperately trying to understand the different terminology, I found myself asking a lot of questions of the doctors and nurses.

During this brief experience I learnt that no question is too silly to ask. At no time should you hold back from questioning the doctor or nurse because you think it's bothering them. With an onslaught of medical jargon, you need to be sure you understand what they are telling you. Take notes if you can, and have a friend or family member with you as a second ear.

Ensure you are heard; advocate for yourself. Be that squeaky wheel, because at the end of the day, we have but one life, and when having to deal with this horrendous disease you want to make sure you are under the best of care and have tried every available treatment, or at least have the information to make an educated decision.

How did this experience affect me? My life is forever changed since my brother died, as understandably, a piece of me is missing. To find a positive is difficult but I am now far more aware of the needs of families going through similar experiences. I have since been able to raise awareness and funds for oesophageal cancer, and now breast cancer, and have met so many wonderful people in the process.

I have been working with So Brave since that first meeting in 2017 and have designed the last three calendars, a multitude of other marketing collateral, and now this book, to raise awareness and educate young women. I have even made a couple of cakes for one of the launches. We all need to be breast aware and consistent in our self-examinations as research shows that early detection helps save lives.

It's been a privilege to play a small role in a wonderful and desperately needed organisation. I have met many inspirational ambassadors during this time and my life is forever changed because of it. I have read their stories and have been constantly amazed at their strength and courage. The one constant I have found after meeting many of these women, is that a positive mindset is like a super power! Some of the women had finished treatment, some had upcoming surgeries and others were still going through treatment, yet all of them had a fabulous sense of humour and were free with a smile.

I hope you are empowered when you read this book and it helps you to carry on during your own experience with the strength I know is inside you.

♡ *Sharon*

Graphic Designer, So Brave – Australia's Young Women's Breast Cancer Charity

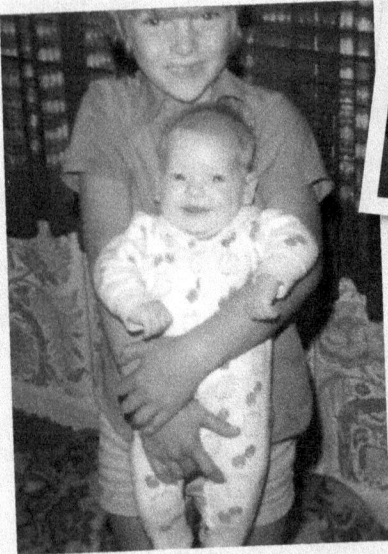

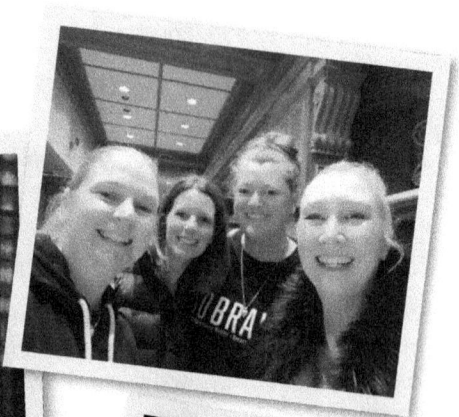

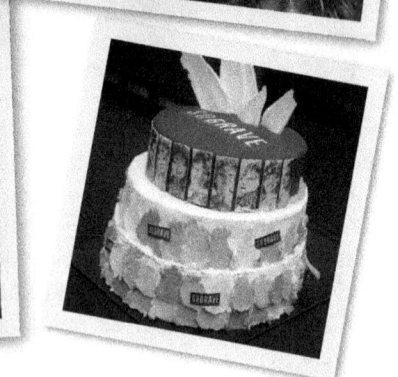

CONTENTS

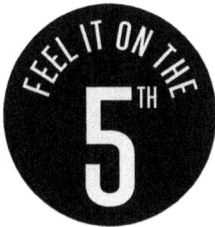

FEEL IT ON THE 5TH

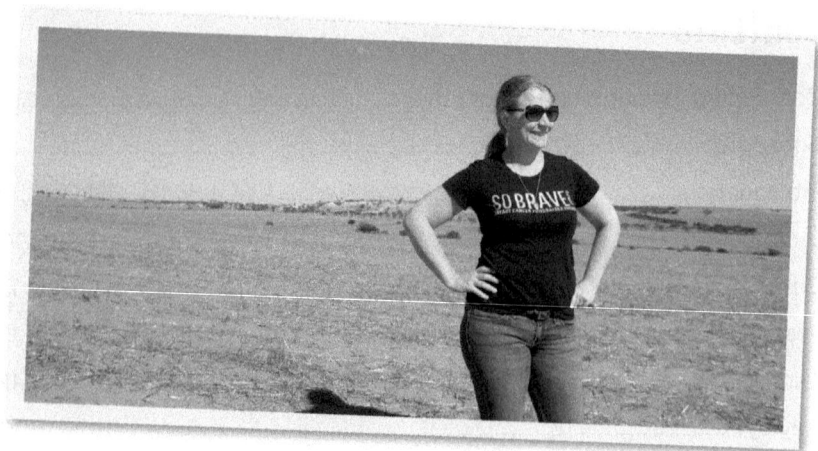
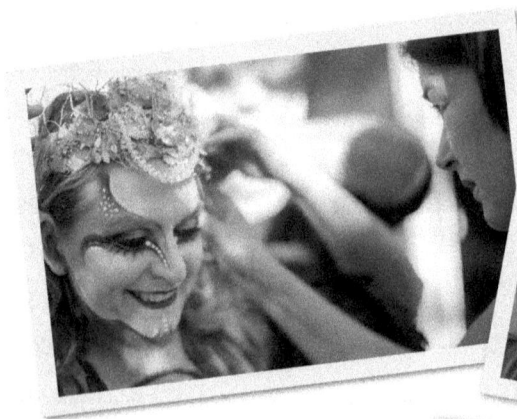
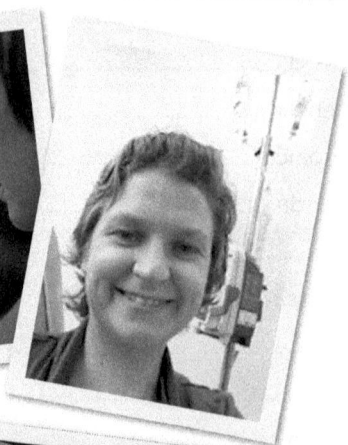
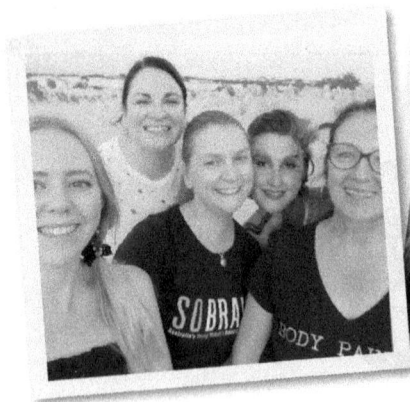
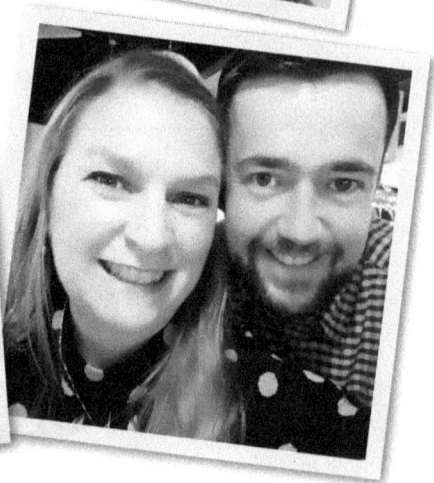

INTRODUCTION

Dear Reader,

This book has come together as a passion project and as a legacy of the work of So Brave since I created it in 2015. So Brave began because I felt quite isolated in a sea of women diagnosed with breast cancer. I was always the youngest in the room at support meetings, my Breast Care nurse didn't know what to tell me about breastfeeding with a newborn and it was really hard on my family. There were many struggles in just getting my diagnosis and these too form the basis of that need for So Brave in the world.

It took me 3 months of talking to specialists and doctors and imaging specialists before I finally got my diagnosis. It took me getting out of my own head and thinking that I was worrying about nothing, especially since I have no family history, I breastfed my first child, I was young, I was pregnant and had no reason to think that this was even possible for me. What I have since found is that my story is not unique. I also discovered that sharing stories became part of my recovery, and that this is true not just for me, but for many women who've been through this. Connecting with women who've been there before helps to heal from your own experience. It provides community, and it allows you to find women you can relate to.

The stories in this book are real and raw, and there's no sugar-coating any of the realities that these women face as young breast cancer survivors. It's been written like that to provide you, our dear reader, with a true account of what it is like to hear those fated words 'you have breast cancer'. It's been written like that to provide you with some hope that there are better days ahead, that just like these brave young women, you too are strong and will get through this horrible ordeal.

We hope you share this with the women in your life and that it inspires you on those grey days.

You're stronger than you know.

♡ *Rachelle*

Founder, So Brave – Australia's Young Women's Breast Cancer Charity

EMMA

To my dear friend,

Well WELCOME!!! Welcome to the club that you never thought you would be a part of, but once you're in it, you make friends, fight demons and conquer cancer.

If you have just been diagnosed, I can imagine, if it's anything like me, you're probably scared, confused, sad, angry and so many more emotions. BUT that's OKAY. It is so normal to feel a range of emotions because you have just been given the news that you would have never thought would happen to you. So, feel what you need to feel.

There are so many things you need to juggle when you get diagnosed and throughout your treatment. I was 24 when I got diagnosed so there was university, work, family, friends, doctors, specialists... oh the list goes on. It seems so overwhelming.

I found the best way was to make sure you have a diary and write everything down as you go. CHEMO BRAIN is a thing. You honestly forget things and forget what you were about to do and what you were about to say but don't worry, it's normal and it does get better. I made sure I had all my appointments in a diary and in my phone so I didn't forget any. I made sure I either recorded my appointments or you might want to take someone in with you as you are given so much information. Some of it can be missed so if someone's with you, or you record it, you can be reminded.

Dealing with people was the next challenge – family, friends, neighbors, colleagues and strangers all want to help or visit or call and find out how you are and what is happening. It can be so overwhelming. When your loved ones ask what they can do to help, give them something they can do instead of saying nothing. Frozen homemade dinners, babysitting if you have kids, taking you to appointments or dropping in occasionally for a coffee. People want to help and I know at the beginning I didn't want to trouble

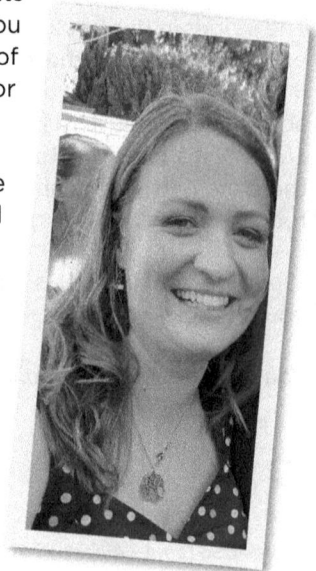

anyone but soon realised these small tasks are actually so exhausting when you're having chemo or surgery and it is such a help.

Also, assign someone close to you to tell people what is happening. My mum knew everything that was happening so when family wanted to know, instead of me getting a billion calls about it, she was able to talk to them instead. I did the same with my best friend. She knew and was able to pass on to others that wanted to know what was happening. At the beginning there is a lot of people around. People are shocked at the news you have cancer and want to help and be there, but over time this dies off, people get busy and go back to their lives, and suddenly it can become quite isolating and lonely, so make sure you reach out. Talk to your loved ones and check in with a counsellor or psychologist every now and then.

I had to make some really tough decisions, I had the BrCa1 gene so I ended up having a mastectomy and partial hysterectomy. There were multiple surgeries, eight rounds of chemotherapy, fertility preservation treatment, and this all involved making choices and it all happened so quickly. My life turned upside down. At the time I just powered on through. It seemed easy at the time. When I wasn't recovering or having chemo I still went to work as a paramedic and powered through. I remember always thinking 'this is ok, I can do this, it's nothing like the movies', but oh was I wrong.

When it all slowed down, chemo finished and I'd recovered from surgery, I fell in a heap. What was my new normal? Will I still have my own family? How will I meet someone when I'm covered in scars, have fake, strange-looking boobs and going through menopause? Trust me, there is no easy fix for these worries, but I am working through them all slowly and with time, I will find my new normal. Life goes on and you jump back into it and you get through each day. I'm lucky to be surrounded by my amazing family and friends which also helps get you through.

The funny thing is, I wouldn't change what has happened. Crazy, I know! I have learnt so much about myself – I can do things that are hard and scary without taking the easy way out. I have learnt so much about the people around me, relationships have grown stronger between family and friends, and I appreciate every single person around me. I have also met some incredible people. I have volunteered for some charity work, SO BRAVE being one of them, and have met some other incredible young people that have gone through breast cancer. I have made friends with these people that I would never have met otherwise. Most importantly,

I have learned that life is a gift, it is short and so valuable. Before this, I took it for granted.

So welcome to the club of Breast Cancer Warriors. I promise you will get through all the hard times and the scary things. One day you will look back on this as a distant time in your life that changed you in many ways, some of them good. Keep going and keep fighting.

Love always

♡ *Emma*

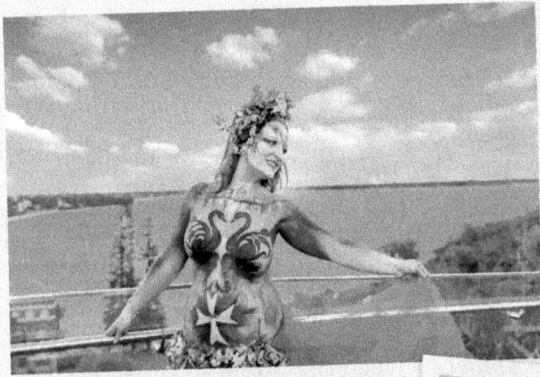

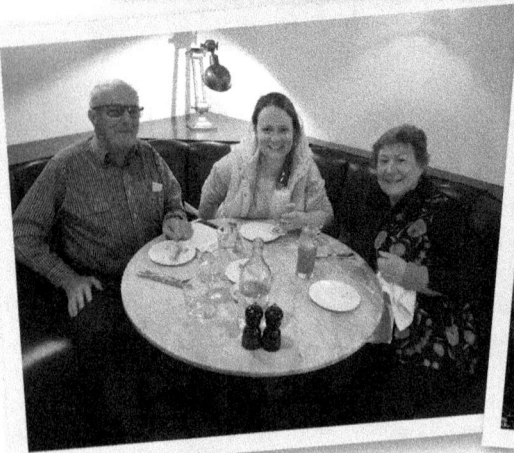

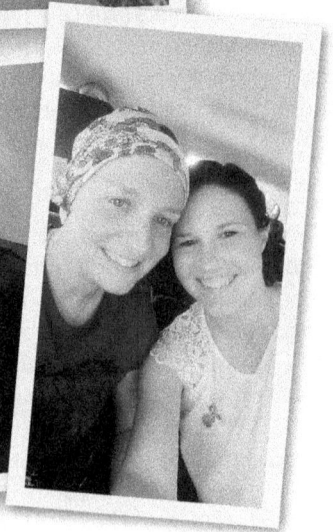

CAROL

Hey,

I know you're in shock. Yesterday you were young, fit and healthy but today you have cancer. It's a strange reality to take in and it probably won't sink in for a few weeks, months or longer! You will be overloaded with information, put through what feels like hundreds of tests, bloods and imaging. Hang in there. At the end of the day, as my own GP said, breast cancer is just a disease that has to be treated. There are thousands of women diagnosed every year and very well established treatments. Just try to breathe!

Make sure you take someone with you to absorb some of the information. Take time to consider your options, especially if and when it comes to reconstruction. Everyone is different and there is no right or wrong. Everyone has their opinions but make sure you listen to your gut.

You'll find that treatment wise you won't have much control, you can only control your mindset and attitude. Let your Oncologist do their job and you just get on with it. My favorite saying throughout my treatment was "you never know how strong you are until being strong is the only choice you have". You didn't choose this, but now it's happened you have no choice but to face it.

Chemo is not as bad as you think it'll be, but if you have a rigorous schedule or thin veins look into getting a port, they are fantastic! They sit just under the skin and make chemo so much quicker and easier because the nurses don't have to find a vein.

The best advice I got was "be selfish". Look after yourself and ask for help. Do whatever you need to do; scream, cry, sit quietly alone, nap! If your body feels like it then you probably need it, but also try and stay busy when you can.

I feel for everyone diagnosed with cancer, it's a crappy club that no one wants to join, but focus on the positives. Don't underestimate the power of connecting with someone who is going through the same thing as you. There are communities on social media and through organisations like So Brave, Cancer Council and Mummy's Wish. Don't be afraid to reach out. It sounds crazy but I've made lifelong friends as a result of my cancer.

If you have children there are charities who specialise and can give you advice on how to approach your diagnosis and discuss it with your kids. I was blown away by all the help that's out there.

I'm currently traveling Australia in a caravan with my family! Having cancer under 40 shook us to the core and made us reassess what we really want out of life. I'm not saying this is the path you should also take but I want you to know there is life after cancer. It might not be the same or where you expected to be but it's yours!

Have faith, you've got this.

♡ Carol

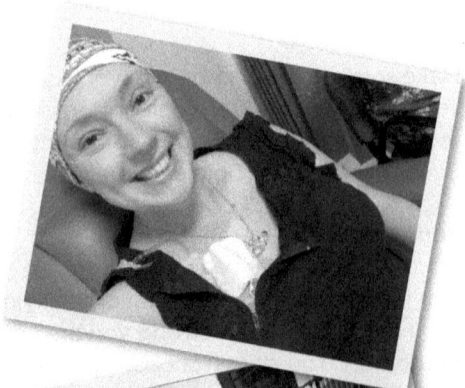
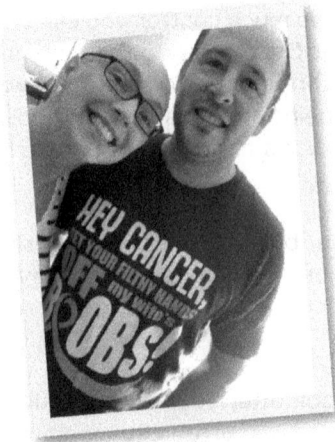
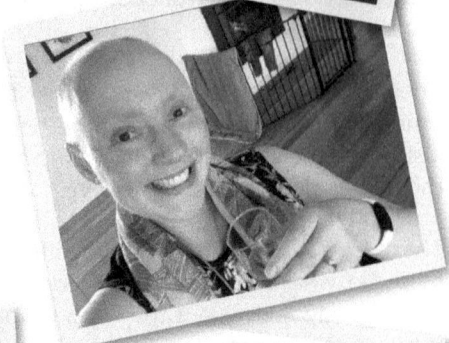
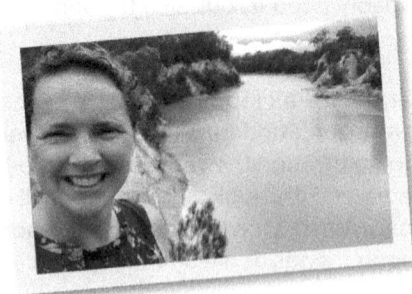
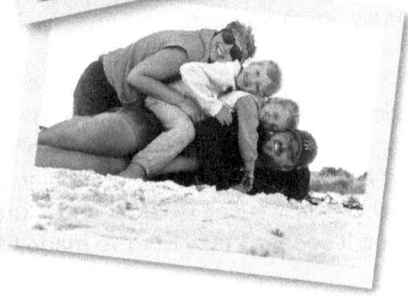

JESS W

Beautiful Human,

I wish that you didn't have to read this. I have been in your shoes and I am alive and well. You can get to the place I am in too. Trust me, I speak the truth.

Life is tough and I know this is something that you never would have chosen to happen to you. This can be a gift or a curse, the choice is yours. This hand you have been dealt is unfair. No one will dispute that, however, the universe does not give us things we cannot handle and you have got this. I wanted you to know there are many of us out there in a similar situation – you are not alone.

We are here for you whenever you need, just reach out and we will be there to support you. If you feel like you don't know anyone yet, and you can't, then reading this will be a start.

The next year will be one of the hardest yet, but will be an investment for your life. This is not the end. It is the beginning.

Listen to your body, it is not fighting against you, it is speaking to you and now is the time to hear it and to respond with what it is so desperate for you to hear – love me, care for me, look after me.

Self-compassion is key at this time as is loving kindness and taking care of yourself.

Self-love is a long hard journey that takes time and this is the beginning of this path for you, where you get to make a choice to surrender, surrender to the care, love and respect deep down, you have for yourself.

If you are asking why this is happening to you, there is no real answer and the question of why will plague you if you continue to ask it. This is one of those situations that simply just is, and the only way out, is through.

Look forward and focus on the small wins, as well as taking one day at a time, will get you through. This is pain manifested. It is stress and trauma and negative energy that is literally eating you alive. The way to heal it is to know it, build a relationship with it and allow it to be seen in order for it to heal.

Feel it to heal it.

Breathe clean air.

Spend time with people that fill you with joy.

Eat foods that nourish you.

Hydrate your soul with goodness.

Change.

Hold yourself up and know that you are worthy, worthy of love, worthy of this life and worthy of the light inside you that you have dimmed.

Call on that light to help you heal.

You are loved. You are light.

I am here for you.

It is time.

Time to heal.

♡ *Jess*

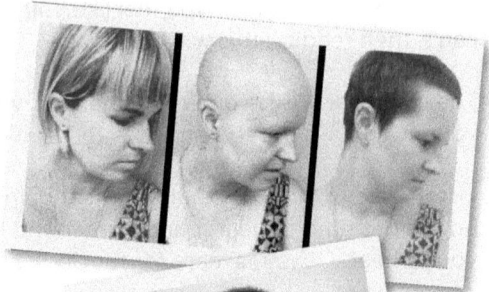

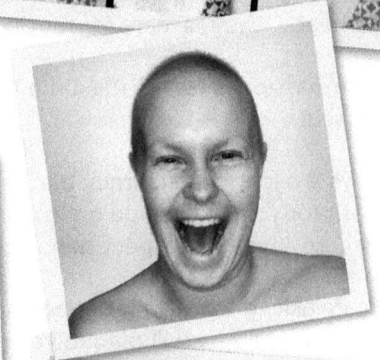

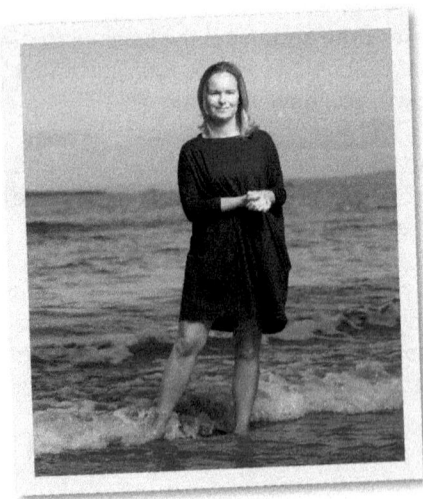

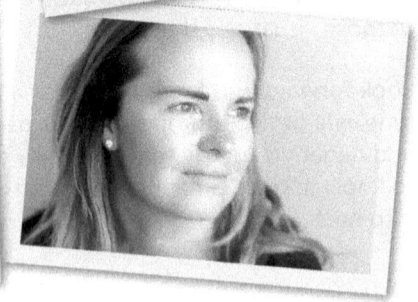

SAM

Dear Sister,

As you read this letter, let me be a rock for you to stand on. If you are anything like me at diagnosis, the ground will have been ripped from beneath your feet. As I started to write this letter, I wanted to share my story, however as I got to the second page, I was nowhere near half way so I'm starting again in the attempt of sharing what has helped me so far on my roller coaster ride.

When I first found out I had breast cancer, my immediate thought was of my Grandma who had died from it. I thought 'How could I have an aggressive breast cancer when I'm only thirty-three? I'm too young to have this!' I found the lump in my right breast after completing a run along the beautiful coast. I was young, fit, healthy and happy. I kept thinking 'If I hadn't checked... if it wasn't for my Grandma I would never had been aware...'. I will be forever grateful to my Grandma. I was young when she passed but I feel her standing with me today, even if we never met. She is always by my side.

I had been following a lady on Instagram, around my age, initially because she was a part of the kelpie owner community – I have a beautiful kelpie, Sheba who has literally been like a mental health nurse. Dogs are amazing! A year ago, I followed her story through pictures of her lying on her couch with no hair, in a hospital bed and with her kelpie snuggled in to her side. She had been diagnosed with breast cancer and had to go through chemotherapy before having a bilateral mastectomy and reconstruction. I can remember thinking how brave she was and how she could make light of a situation.

When I felt the lump in my right breast, she was my first port of call. I can remember writing my first email to her, thinking that I may be overstepping the Instagram friendship line. When she replied, she literally became my hero. She answered my thousand, if not more, questions and sent me a beautiful package from MooGoo (amazing product for your skin during radiotherapy). After lots of conversations and advice, we met in Bondi when I travelled with my sister, which was like meeting an old buddy. She brought her kelpie, Ralphie along and we had a great chat over lunch, overlooking Bondi Beach, discussing different boob reconstructions, what helps make your hair grow back, and of course, kelpies. If I can recommend anything to help ladies who have just been diagnosed, it is to communicate with others who have been through the same. It literally saved my sanity to ask any question, any time of day and night, and to have that safety net of somebody who understands through their own experience.

Before my diagnosis, I could laugh at myself if I made mistakes or if I did something silly. Now, I am constantly laughing at myself with the things I find myself doing. I've found myself putting TV remotes in the freezer, freaked out because I'd 'lost' my mobile while speaking to my sister on my mobile and there's that time when my fake boob fell out and landed on my foot at the gym! That's just to name a few things that I've done since having chemotherapy. Sure, chemotherapy can mess up your thinking and can sometimes affect your memory but hey, it is part of a process where the aim is to save your life. I was told to think of the chemotherapy drugs as racing horses sprinting through my veins, destroying anything threatening in their path. This visual image helped me immensely. I hope it helps you too.

After chemotherapy, I needed radiotherapy as I had one node out of nine involved. The nurses were beautiful, and it was nothing compared to chemotherapy. I made sure I treated myself to a nice coffee every day and made time to sit in the garden. I also caught up with my sister on her days off where we could sit and talk. Another important thing to remember is to communicate. Even if it's over a coffee or a nice walk with a loved one or a friend. You need to talk, don't let your thoughts fill your head to the point where you begin to think dark thoughts. Air them and let them out into the sunshine where they can be heard.

I am now on anti-hormone drugs which cause a forced menopause. I now experience daily 'personal summers' aka hot flushes. It's like a personal heating system. I will be meeting with my breast surgeon to discuss having another mastectomy. It is a personal choice. I have gained a LOT of respect for people and their choices, and I am going to stay 'flat' for a period before deciding on reconstruction. I look at my body now, after years of complaining of my big bum, big thighs and a tummy and see something amazing. My body has had a breast amputated, another one to come off, has been poisoned, radiated and put into forced menopause and she's still strong and energetic. My body, your body, is amazing.

So, remember, talk to your fellow sisters, imagine those horses racing through your veins, sit in the sunshine and love you for being you. If I could, I would give you a warm hug and drink hot chocolate with you. Maybe one day, we will meet, and we can have that hot chocolate.

Remember, YOU are amazing, find your fire and use it.

♡ Sam

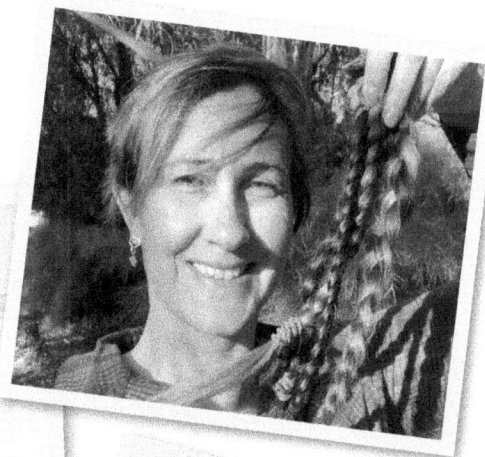

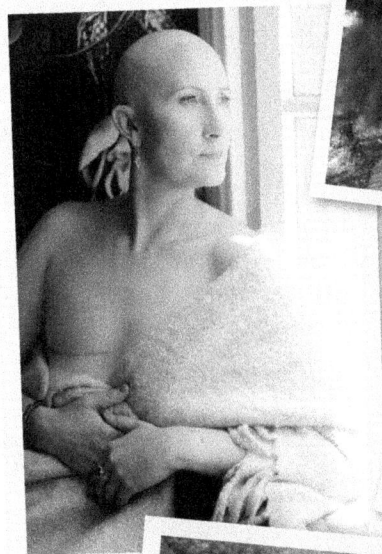

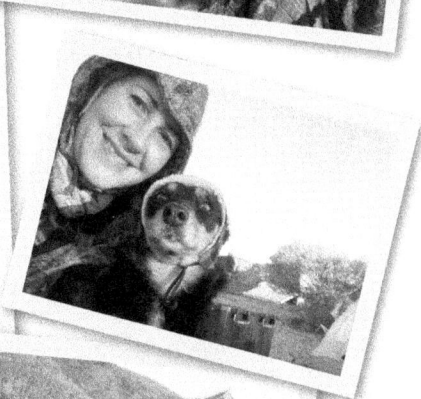

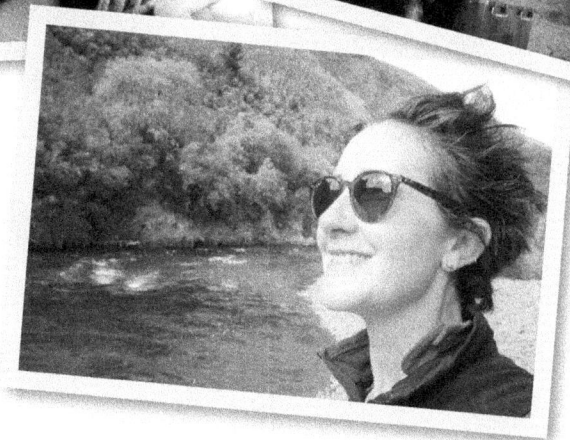

HAYLEY

Dear friend,

I know this may feel so big right now that you can barely process it.

It may feel like you can't deal with this, or that it's not real and I'm so sorry that you are in this position.

I'll tell you right now, there are tough times ahead, but I'll also tell you this... you are tough.

Tougher than you may ever have realised.

There are physical factors you'll have to deal with now. Physical scars along with the emotional ones.

I need you to have faith, faith in your own strength, faith in your own ability to heal and thrive, but also that the universe has your back and it will always be supporting you with love.

Take time to rest, to look after yourself, to nurture not only your body but your soul. Do things that fill you with happiness, spend time with those you love. Don't waste time on negative people or people who crush your energy. Now is the time to focus on all your needs.

This will change you and while you may not be able to see any kind of silver lining right now, look for the love around you and love is all you'll ever need. Love will help you through this.

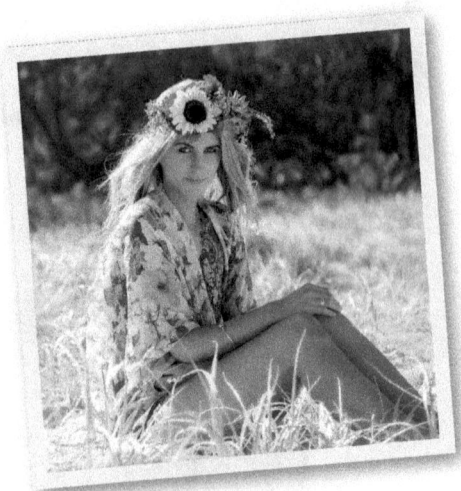

♡ Hayley

SUE

Hi there love,

I'm so sorry to hear of your cancer news. You are probably feeling overwhelmed and like it's a little unreal. So just a quick note to say I'm thinking of you.

Some people like to hear a bit of what might be in front of them. I was a bit like a sponge, wanting to know everything, so I'll share a bit of what my road so far has brought and taught me.

Not sure if you're going to head for surgery, chemo, radiation, or all three. I can tell you a bit about the first two, take all or nothing on board. It's not going to be the same for you and you don't necessarily need to hear it right now. Read it later if you like, or just say "thanks Sue but I need to figure this out alone" and that's ok.

Breast cancer covers such a wide range and severity of disease, I really hope in your case, as in mine, they have caught it early and have found it's a less aggressive type. Regardless, all treatments have come so far, I think if you had to get this blasted c- disease, then possibly breast cancer is one of the best and well-researched.

I'm almost four months in from initial diagnosis, and it's all gone very quick. Three surgeries ending in a mastectomy before Christmas, and now just completed my second chemo treatment. I wasn't too wrapped up in losing the breast, better that than a hand or leg, but it is a bit confronting and certainly a bother leaving the house and remembering a breast form all the time. I couldn't have reconstruction straight away but it's something I plan on post chemo.

Chemo, chemo, chemo. Where to begin? You may not need it so that's the first thing. If the cancer has spread to more than the sentinel nodes you probably will. It's not the descent into hell that I had feared, and that in the early days of chemotherapy, it probably was. I get tired, drained and listless, aches and pains, a bit of nausea and a cycle of constipation-diarrhoea-constipation. As a friend said to me before I started, "I'm going to be honest, it's going to suck". It does but it's not insurmountable. You can function, and it gets a bit better every day past the treatment day. I know some people work through chemo and I don't know how they do it. If you have any capacity to take some time off work, then do it. I'm using income protection and we're taking a hit financially, but I simply couldn't work, my mind and emotions aren't clear enough. What's more, I'm currently shedding hair everywhere! My cereal this morning, keyboard right now; that's not something I need at work. Consider work from home options perhaps, if you need to work and if your work is amenable?

Two other points of advice, then I'm done.

- Take all the help offered. Don't feel unworthy or a burden. There are a lot of cancer support groups that provide practical support and grab help from family and friends with both hands.

- How you deal with this is going to be different from everyone else, but it's all valid and all ok. Don't feel guilty about depression or fatigue or wanting to hide away for a bit. On the other hand, if you want to go out and celebrate and get on with life as normal, that's also good. Whatever your coping mechanism is, don't judge yourself, just cope. You will get through it; we both will.

Sending you love and a soft hug and a tear, will speak soon,

♡ Sue

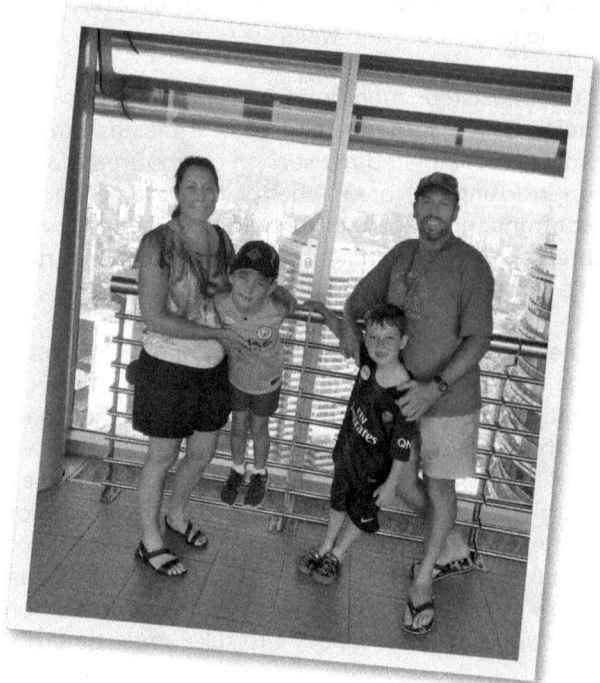

JESS B

Dear sweatheart,

I am sorry that you have to read this and I had to write it, but it is important to know that you are not alone on this journey. You might feel lost like I did. Lost between your old life, which vanished overnight, as you are plunged into this new world. You did not ask for this, and have every right to struggle to adapt to it. It's okay not to be okay. To face the reality that you will need to rely heavily on others, to give in to the pain, and want or need to cry, scream or run at the severity of all of this. You will probably feel drained mentally, physically, and emotionally, but you will push on like you always do. Put one foot in front of the other, like there is no other way. But just try to remember, you are not alone.

When I was diagnosed and whilst I was undergoing treatment for breast cancer, well intentioned people often reminded me that "these days most people survive breast cancer" and "breast cancer charities get so much money because of its pink marketing". These are common statements when it comes to breast cancer, but are in fact misconceptions about the type of breast cancer that I was diagnosed with. You might find that some people do not know what to say, say the wrong thing or say nothing at all. Try not to take this too personally as you are probably the youngest person they know who has cancer.

I was diagnosed with breast cancer after a biopsy on my 30th birthday. Doctors always test for three different clinical markers: estrogen receptor, progesterone receptor and human epidermal growth factor receptor. The results would determine what kind of treatment I would receive. My cancer was negative to these three receptors and because of that I was diagnosed with triple negative breast cancer. Hang on to whatever positive news you get – you are young and a fighter. It's important to remember that they found it at all and that you will give this thing everything you have got until it packs its bags and leaves its temporary host.

After my tumour was removed, I went through a round of IVF. Following this, the only treatment available to me was intensive chemotherapy, which is gruelling and has no guarantee of success. To finish, a bilateral mastectomy, which crushed my body image and future hopes of breast feeding. But, my health had to come first or there would be no future at all. You will be buffeted with shock after shock. Then will come the waves of decisions, specialist after specialist, waiting room after waiting room, all compounded by the upending of your well-laid plans.

You need to trust your treatment team, and if you are safe and being treated appropriately, you will be given the time and space to get as much information as you can and not feel like you need to rush into decisions immediately. Try to control what decisions you can make. For me this was things like shaving my head when I wanted, and choosing the support team I wanted around me.

Whilst my prognosis is good, and I am on my way to getting back to "normal" life, I don't like to use the words "survivor" or "in remission". Yes, I had cancer and yes, it happened to me, but no, it is not a part of who I am. Like any other traumatic experience in life, you get through it. Try to learn from it and then move forward.

♡ *Jess*

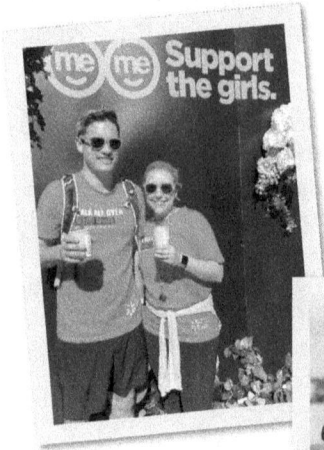

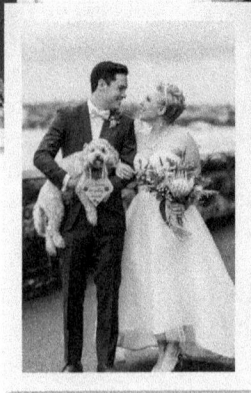

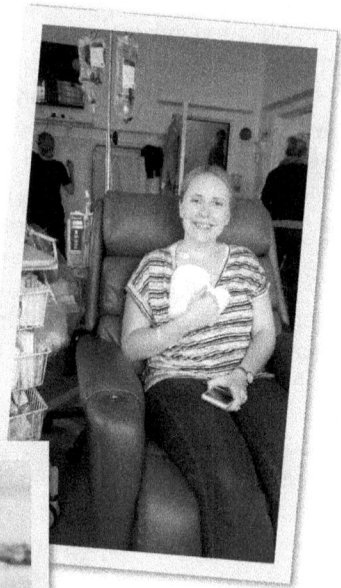

MICHELLE

Beautiful girl,

You have been given the hardest news and right now I am sure you have so many emotions. These are emotions that only you will understand and for this reason, take time to be kind to yourself.

Surround yourself with family, friends and loved ones that support you, care for you and know when to let you have your own space to cry and mourn if you need to.

Throughout our lives we have many friends. Some will stay with you for a lifetime and many will come and go. This is life. No one is perfect and sometimes people make poor choices. If you have been the best friend you can be and certain friends don't support you through this, let them go. Don't make it about you, you know you are a good person. Accept the ones you want to accept, move on from those that don't. You won't look back I promise.

Love your body. Your body has been through so much and is fighting to keep you alive. You may need surgery, chemo or radiation and with this, your body will change. Your body DOES NOT define you, nor does it allow people the right to pass judgement on you. Remember you are beautiful inside and out.

Your personal relationships and love life will be tested. You CANNOT change people. It doesn't matter if your partner is male or female, if they care about you, they will support you 100% regardless. If your partner doesn't speak to you with empathy, listen to your fears and hold you when you're scared, ask yourself why? This is the time you need to focus on you. Make sure the person beside you has your back. NEVER allow someone to put you down. NEVER allow anyone to question who you are. And NEVER EVER allow someone to make you feel less than you are worth. If you need to do this without them, you will be ok.

Know that you are in charge of you and you can choose to feel any way you want to. It takes work to do this, so don't let the thought monsters control you. DO NOT accept defeat, just keeping working at it one day at a time. Don't believe the negative thoughts and feelings that sometimes pop into your head, they aren't true. Be angry, be sad... but be honest with your feelings and go back and read all of this again.

You are stronger than you realise and braver than you know.

You've got this!

Your sister,

♡ *Michelle*

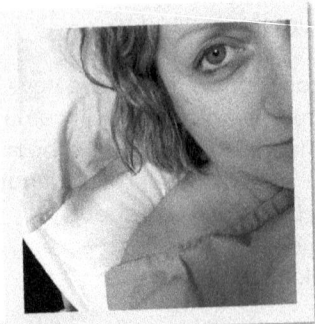

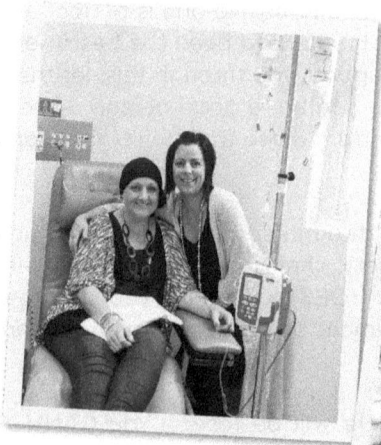

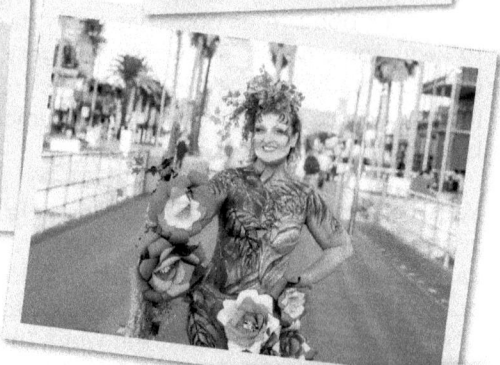

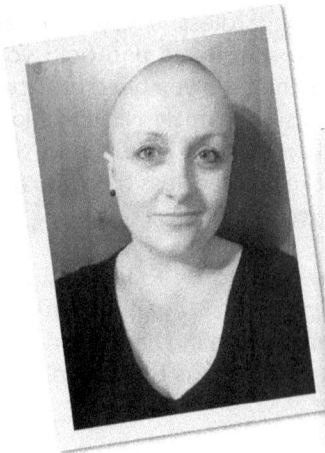

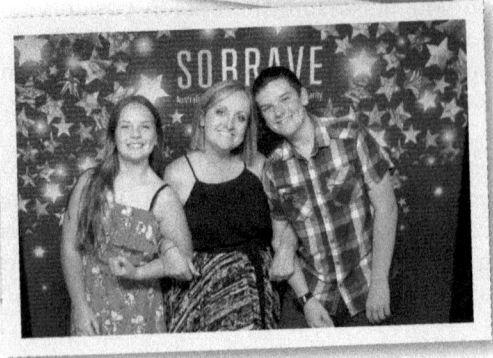

VERONICA

Dear You,

Firstly, let me say, I'm sorry you are going through this difficult period! Please know that there will always be a loving tribe out there to support you. It's an exclusive club no one joins willingly, but once you're in it you will find friendships like no other you've ever experienced.

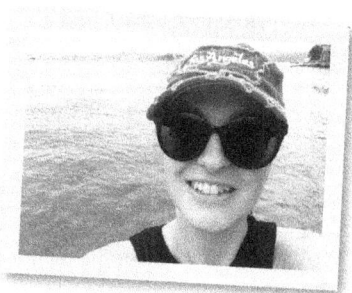

I was 40 years old when I was diagnosed with HER2+ breast cancer, which had spread to the lymph nodes in my armpit. At the time of my diagnosis, we had only been married 18 months and had undergone 2 IVF attempts, which sadly were unsuccessful.

Four years on, all treatment and breast reconstruction complete, I often look back and reflect... as hard as the last 4 years have been, they have also been some of the happiest and full of blessings. This may be hard to believe when you're in the midst of diagnosis and various forms of challenging treatments. Personally, I have used this time for introspection and work through what I want out of life going forward.

I won't lie, it's not an easy journey and it impacts your relationships; it has certainly impacted our marriage, our intimacy and the dreams we had for our future. As a couple we're committed to working through it together, and reimagine what the future might look like for us. Our family picture isn't what we had imagined, but it's a loving family nevertheless.

I do feel like I have been given a second chance at life, and although cancer is often at the back of my mind I don't always think about it... heck there are days I almost forget it happened!!!

I focus on the work I want to do, and the impact I want to have on the world. I'm now dedicating time to project and business ideas as well as volunteering. Life is more rewarding these days.

There will always be scares, and at those times I allow myself to be vulnerable and seek the help I need to navigate those fearful moments... I'm now really good at asking for help and I would encourage you all to do the same.

If I were to share some guidance on what I have found helpful to me, and I hope it may prove to be helpful to you all my dear sisters, it is this:

- When possible, embrace a positive/grateful mindset.

- Allow yourself to be vulnerable and cared for.

- Be open to the wondrous connections that will come your way. I have experienced amazingly sincere connections whilst on this journey.

- Keep communication channels open in your relationships. Although it can be incredibly frustrating that "others" won't fully understand what we're going through, it is important to keep our loved one's part of our journey.

- And lastly, but certainly not least – nurture yourself! Now is your time to give yourself everything you need spiritually, emotionally and physically. Listen to your body, it'll tell you what it needs.

I came across this quote from Paulo Coelho: "Not all storms come to disrupt your life, some come to clear your path". I honestly believe this and once I'd had my surgery to remove the cancer, I worked hard to adopt a positive mindset. It has meant a world of difference for me in my journey.

I wish you all the very best for your treatments, recovery and future health. I sincerely mean it when I say, feel free to reach out to me should you ever need to. You don't need to walk this road alone.

♡ Veronica

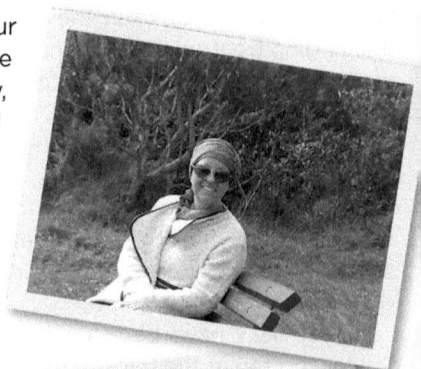

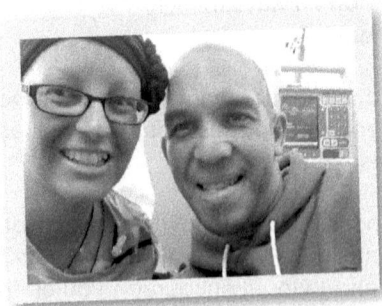

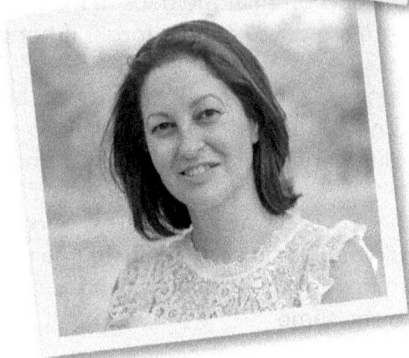

BELINDA

To my new-found Pink Sister,

What a terrible shock you have just had, finding out about your breast cancer diagnosis. Even if you had entertained the possibility that you would hear bad news, nothing quite prepares you for actually hearing the news that you have cancer. Hearing those words is incredibly confronting and frightening.

It is a time of complete, raw emotion. I personally found it extremely helpful, comforting and reassuring to hear of others' experiences. So I am here to share with you a part of my story.

I was diagnosed in July 2018 at age 38. At the time of diagnosis my two boys were 4 years old and 9 months old.

I thought I would share with you my chemotherapy path.

I had chemotherapy post-surgery. I had a bilateral mastectomy with bilateral axillary clearance. The cancer was a lot more extensive than first thought, and I do wonder that if the extent of it had been picked up on scans, possibly the decision may have been to have chemotherapy prior to surgery. My cancer was put at Stage 3c when the pathology results came back.

The day I met my oncologist, I took my husband and my best friend with me. My oncologist is an interesting fellow and the complete opposite to my warm, friendly breast surgeon. He is by no means rude and horrible, just very straight to the point with a sarcastic sense of humour.

I was feeling quite scared and fragile, and I was extremely grateful to have the support with me. I was told in the appointment that I would be having 2 types of chemotherapy. The first lot is called AC (Adriamycin and Cyclophosphamide), which is a combination of two chemotherapies. It is usually given once every 3 weeks for 12 weeks. However, I was to receive this in a Dose Dense form (once every 2 weeks over 8 weeks). When it is given dose dense, there is less time for the body cells to recover, hence, making the chemotherapy more effective, however, it has a much greater impact on the body as there is also less time for the healthy cells to recover. The second lot would be called Paclitaxol and be given weekly over the course of 12 weeks.

My oncologist explained that this would absolutely exhaust me. He also explained that I would lose all my hair, however, I could choose to attend his private hospital cancer clinic and use the 'cold cap' if I wanted to. This could possibly prevent the loss of all my head hair and it wasn't going to leave me out of pocket with my health insurance, so I decided to give it a go.

I was super nervous the day that chemo was kicking off. I'm sure everyone is for their first treatment. The nurses at the cancer centre were fabulous. Very informative, but compassionate and caring too. My husband came with me for my first treatment. Due to using the cold cap, the day took a good 5 to 6 hours. This is due to needing to cool the scalp prior to and after the chemotherapy is given. The AC usually takes around 2 to 2.5 hours. So it made for a long day and a very cold head. The cold cap basically cools all your hair follicles in an attempt to prevent hair loss. The Cap cools your head to around 3-5 degrees from memory. Yes, it is super cold, gives you an ice-cream headache and blankets are required.

I was super nervous that the chemotherapy would make me feel sick straight away. To my surprise, I just felt normal. I had it given through a port catheter (which had been inserted the week before to my upper left chest area). Due to my bilateral axillary clearance, it was better practice to use a port for me and therefore decrease my risk of lymphoedema occurring.

The following day after my first session I still felt ok. I was surprised. I had been given an injection to self-administer that afternoon. It is called Neulasta and it is to boost the body's white blood cells to try and keep the immune system functioning.

The following morning (day 2 post chemo) I felt dreadful. I had been warned that this injection could cause bone pain. Well, it certainly did for me. It felt like my entire body was bruised. This lasted a good 24-48 hours and occurred each time I used this medication. I used Paracetamol to help me with this and would hibernate away for a day. With each dose of the AC chemo I became more tired, had bouts of nausea and lost my sense of taste.

I lost a large amount of my hair after the second AC dose. I continued using the cold cap, but after my final AC dose, I was very close to packing it in. My head had become so sensitive, I felt horrible and was probably the closest I had ever been to feeling depressed. However, I had two young children who still wanted their mum. I really feel that this kept pushing me forward and I tried to go about daily chores and activities as best as possible.

I had my husband or a friend come with me to each of the AC chemo sessions, mainly as I wasn't sure how I would be driving myself home, but also for some company.

When the time came to start the weekly Paclitaxal chemotherapy, I had heightened anxiety as I wasn't quite sure if I could face another 12 weeks of doing this to my body. The Paclitaxal only takes an hour, so my cold cap session was basically cut in half. I decided to keep on with the cold cap, knowing I could stop at any time. I had kept around 40-50 percent of my hair by this stage.

Your blood tests are regularly checked throughout having chemotherapy. My second week in to the Paclitaxal, my Haemoglobin levels had dropped to 83, and had been dropping consistently. I was anaemic and felt like it too. The decision was made to give me a blood transfusion. I was hesitant to begin with, but my exhaustion levels were becoming difficult to manage. It took a number of weeks to have good effect, but when it did, it greatly improved my energy levels and my determination to get through this stage of treatment.

Thankfully for me, the weekly chemo was easy. My body coped with it well. I ended up driving myself to and from the hospital for the last 7 weeks. My hair started to grow back. I didn't need to give myself any more Neulasta injections, so no more bone pain. I did have to use ice packs to my hands and feet to try and ward off peripheral neuropathy. This seems to be very dependent on your oncologist's beliefs. I do have some mild neuropathy to my right foot, but I seem to have come away with minimal issues.

A few things I took with me during the chemo sessions were, audio books, downloaded Netflix shows, magazines and sometimes I would sleep. I would take a large bottle of water with one of the cold Lipton tea infusers to add some flavour and would also take eucalyptus drops to suck on. Strange, but I think because they had a strong flavour it helped.

I had an amazing network of supportive friends and family who stepped up to help us out with childcare and meals throughout my chemotherapy experience. We had meals dropped off to us 3 times per week. I had a cleaner paid for by some of my aunts and uncles and loads of messages to check in on our family. Having so much love and support really helped us to keep strong.

I could keep on going, however I am going to stop myself here. I can only hope that by me sharing this, you are able to gain some insight and reduce any anxiety you may have. Yes, it is a long 5 to 6 months, but you will get through this as so many before you have, and you will likely surprise yourself with the willpower you have to KEEP ON GOING.

Loads of Love and Hugs to you,

♡ *Belinda*

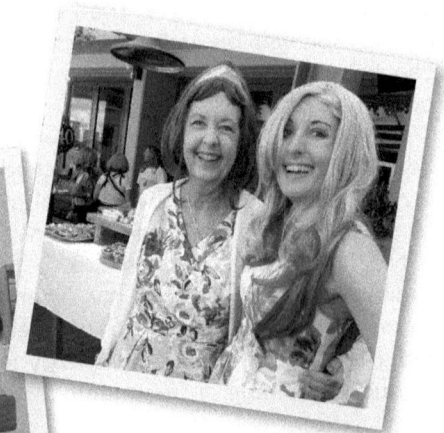

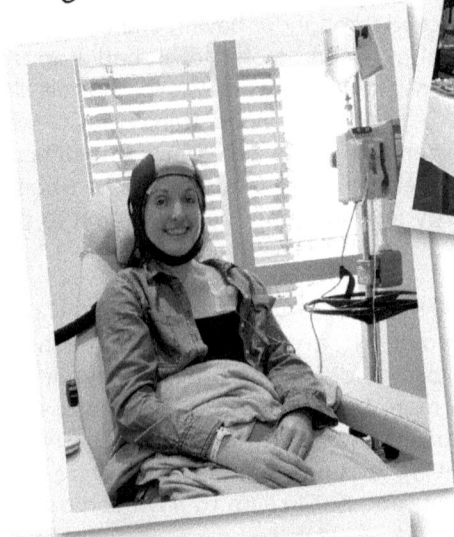

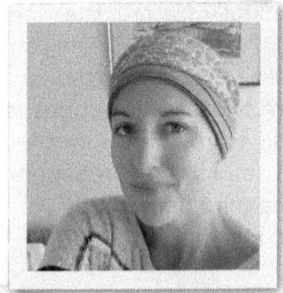

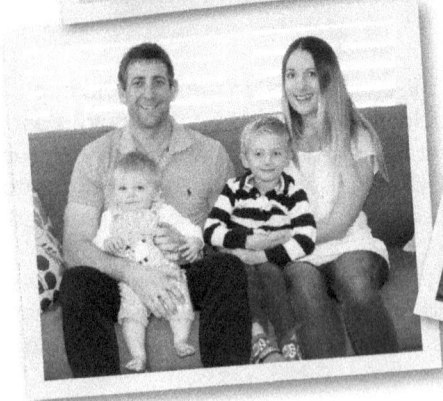

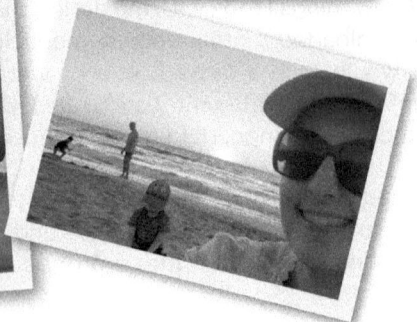

TINA

Dear Gorgeous Girl,

There are not enough words to say I'm sorry you have been diagnosed with this bastard of a disease. So, I will simply say I'm sorry. I hope there are people in your life for the times when you need them – those 2am calls to cry or just chat, a walk when you can, a good laugh, wig shopping, or who can drive you to appointments.

I was you 12 years ago in April 2008. The diagnosis came out of left-field and hit me like a tonne of bricks. I had no family history, I was fit and young (37 – and hey, young women don't get breast cancer, or so we are told!).

I chose to deal with the diagnosis and treatment with humour. It is what helped me get through the days. I found myself not working for the first time as I took a leave of absence from work and honestly, I was bored in the beginning. Later, I was too tired to be bored...

I do want to say this to you. You can get through this. It won't be easy and the emotions will be a roller-coaster. Just go along with it. Find your circle who will be there for you and won't judge you. Yep, that will happen – judgement. Many people will have opinions. Opinions on why you were diagnosed – remember that cake you had? Yep, it was because of that and the nasty sugars... Opinions on the treatment you have chosen to move forward with... some will believe natural remedies are the way to go and let you know their strong thoughts on the pharmaceutical industry conspiracy. Others will insist modern western medicine is what you should do. Darling, choose what you feel comfortable with. There will be opinions on your fertility and if you should choose to freeze your eggs. Some will be supportive and some won't. The judgement and opinions will be endless. One more thing – DO NOT GOOGLE. If you do google, promise me you will only visit reputable sites such as So Brave, NBCF, BCNA, McGrath Foundation, or Cancer Australia.

Treatment will be tough, but do-able. I found having someone I can laugh with during treatment was helpful. I also found after each treatment, recovery took a tad longer. I just went with it. Everyone has a different experience with chemo. I found it was not too bad, just not great. I became more tired with each cycle. Take the meds. Please, please take the meds. I found I was nauseous and knew I would be worse without the meds. Take the meds – there you go, that's my opinion.

After treatment, I wanted to go back to normal. The thing is my normal no longer existed. I was a new person and the goal posts had shifted within me. I did learn that if treatment was six months, give yourself 12 months to recover. You will still be tired. Don't push yourself too hard. You and

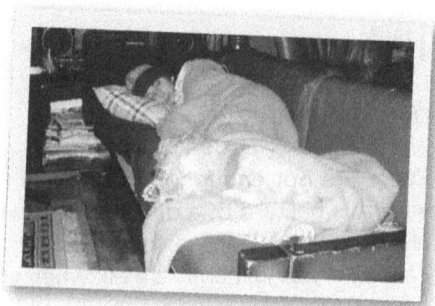

your amazing body have gone through hardcore diagnosis, surgery and treatment. Take it one step at a time. Maybe visit a physio who specialises in post breast cancer rehab, or look into Encore which is a great program for women who had breast cancer surgery and truly helps with their arm mobility.

Tamoxifen! Ahhhh Tamoxfen! Otherwise known as Tamoxibitch. I don't know if you will be prescribed this medication. It will depend on your pathology results. I was prescribed Tamoxibitch and honestly, I struggled.

Darling friend, I could go on and on, and this short letter will become a novel and I won't do that to you. You have too much on your plate right now. I am here for you and know I will support you regarding any decision you make, even if I personally don't agree. I will be there, because that's what friends and sisters do, and now we are sisters in scars.

Love always.

♡ Tina

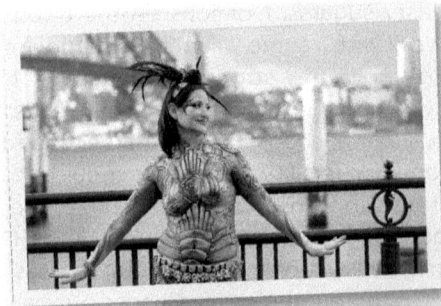

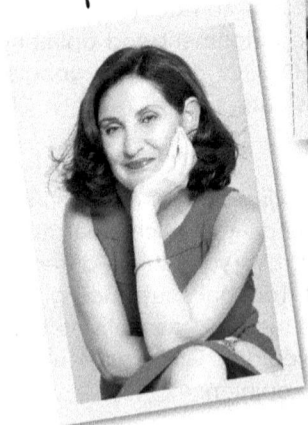

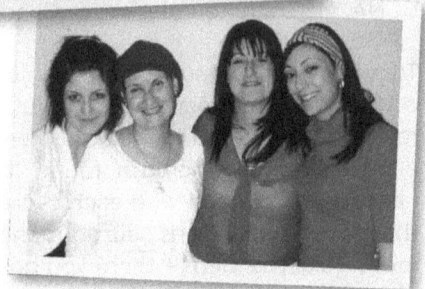

CHELSEA

Dear Cool, Young, Busy, Friendly, Strong, Brave Woman,

Most importantly, it's not as bad as you're imagining it will be. It's not like it is in the movies.

You're about to start chemo – you will not know what to expect and you will Google too much. Acknowledge it, don't go down the Google rabbit hole too often and instead, find some cool people to follow on Instagram, it really does help!

This isn't a letter about feelings, this is what helped me, and some tidbits that might help you. Breast cancer doesn't define you, you probably don't feel sick, you probably don't look sick, you probably were never sick, you probably hate being thought of as being sick. That's good! Although breast cancer is serious and it is one hell of an inconvenience, if the cancer was removed at surgery you might think that you 'had' cancer and now chemo is your 'insurance policy'. If this helps you re-frame how you see yourself, then go for it.

Your people will be shocked, sad & scared... Once they get over the initial shock, they will adapt as quickly as you have. Having your people cheering you on, rather than feeling sad for you, is the best help. Use your village, give people roles and learn to just say 'thank you.' You're allowed to make dark cancer jokes if it helps you cope, humour is ok. You're allowed to have days of 'shit, this sucks' but mostly, you're allowed to rest and do what makes you feel normal.

The scariest part is that first 'chemo' consult and the first infusion. I'll get to this shortly. People our age don't have chemotherapy, it's not like a broken arm or childbirth, it's likely none of your friends have been through it. If you're an information person, then go mad

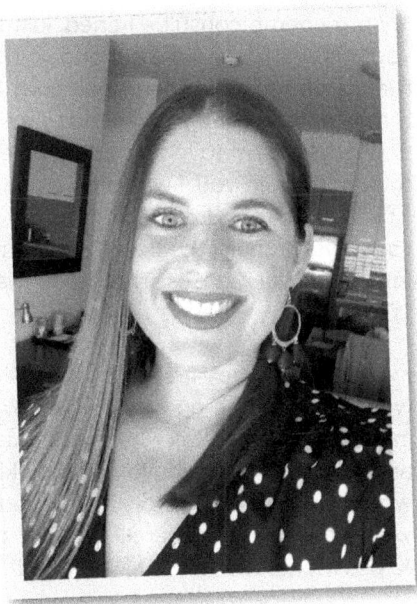

with your Google searches, it satisfies the late night information craving. Learn what sites/forums/Instagram hashtags work for you and stick with them. There's a lot of rubbish out there in internet land, but there's a lot of cool women on Instagram sharing their breast cancer stories. Reach out to them, make a BC friend – they'll 'get it'.

Prep for the worst, then be pleasantly relieved if it's not so bad and you're ok. Stock up on salt mouth washes (I never needed them), buy/hire a wig (I chose never to wear it), gratefully accept gifts of food & care packages, and if you can afford it, outsource anything you can, whether it's a house cleaner (the best), food delivery services or gardening services. Prepare for it whilst you're feeling good.

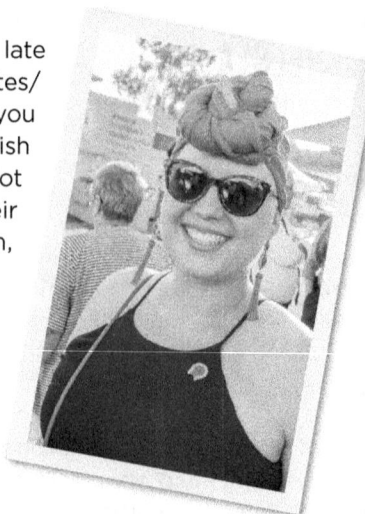

I was lucky enough to have an amazing employer and ample sick & annual leave that I could take the initial rounds off of work – if you have the leave, use it. Get the haircut sorted and work out your 'chemo routine', spend time with friends and keep exercising! The time will come when you don't want to, but until then, keep up your routine.

My pre-chemo consult – I cried, just for minute – even if you're not a crier, you might still cry. Take a friend so they can relay all the info to your other friends and to save them their own Google search. You might be all over the symptoms but your friends aren't. Let them come with you, but feel free to ask them to look it up themselves, rather than repeat to them what the doctor told you. I was prescribed the 4 x fortnightly rounds of AC then 12 x weekly rounds of Taxol regime. The 2 drugs felt massively different. I set myself goals: the 4 x AC then the 12 x weekly Taxol rounds broken up into 4 x 3 week doses. This made the countdown easier and broke up the 20 weeks.

I went alone to my first chemo infusion by choice. Some things you might want to do alone and that's ok. I was lucky enough to have my chemo in the same hospital where I worked so I knew the staff already, I had ample friends in the building, and I knew I could send a text and someone would be there when or if I needed them. Don't feel weird if you don't want an audience. There'll be a lot of talk about symptoms, side effects & pre-medications. You won't get all the symptoms. They might give you anti-nausea medications to take 'if needed' – take them anyway – I was all about the 'just in case' medications and I was never nauseous or felt sick... take the meds. Also, drink water the day before and the days afterwards to plump up your veins and flush out the chemo. Cannulas are ok if you're ok with needles. The oncology nurses are the experts so just try to stay hydrated and calm and your veins will thank you for it. I didn't want a 'port' to make access easier. I was ok with needles and didn't want another 'thing'. I hated being weighed and having my blood pressure taken, but if you chat to the nurses, you can come up with a deal. I weighed myself every second visit towards the end and made the nurses wait till I was comfy and the cannula was in before they did my blood pressure. Compromise, you're in charge!

After my first infusion I met some friends for lunch, I felt quite hyped up from the pre-meds (steroids) and probably some anxiety made me extra talkative. I've never taken a party drug, but it's what I imagine waiting for it to kick in might feel like! I then took my dog for a walk, called my Mum and my Aunty and then went to the gym, easy peasy!

The first 3 days of each of the 4 AC rounds can only be described as a '3 day hangover but without the fun part'. I slept a lot, I took naps throughout the day and found a routine that helped. The steroids suck and make sleeping difficult – take naps. Exercise helps but also makes you feel tired too – take naps and take the low intensity options at the gym. I had rotten headaches. I found the chiropractor really helpful and by round 3 never had another headache.

You might want to have a plan for your hair situation. I had my hairdresser on standby to shave my head once my hair falling out started annoying me. I lasted 2 weeks post first chemo infusion before my hair started to come out after I went for a swim, I was feeling pretty smug that it hadn't started coming out and then, surprise! I was warned it might hurt, it was totally painless. I lasted about 5 days before it got annoying, it was 11am on a Sunday morning when I went for the chop. I didn't want an audience. My cousin came with me and we facetimed another friend (she was given the role of 'hair friend'). I put on bright pink lipstick to make me feel like the focus was away from my hair. My hairdresser was great, no-nonsense, no time to dwell on the occasion. We joked I'd always been low maintenance but this was excessive even for me! By 11.30am my cousin and I were sipping on champagne and sending shaved head selfies to everyone.

I do wonder if being bald is like having a pregnant belly, lots of people will want to touch your head... Swimming feels nice though, swim in the ocean bald at least once! You can get really cool pre-tied hair turbans and you might get really good at tying head scarves. Be creative, wear lipstick and you'll feel better.

You might find you get lots of weird little complaints... the weirdest thing no one told me was the lack of nostril hairs! Your nose might bleed and run uncontrollably. Ask about a nose oil to help prevent nose bleeds and try a room humidifier at night. I also thought having shellac nail polish helped protect my nails. Everyone had a different opinion on this but it helped me, and also made me feel nicer when my nails did discolour towards the end of treatment. Out of sight, out of mind.

As you near the end of chemo, stuff changes again. You might start to feel emotional about being so close to the end, like a kid at Christmas, you might be so excited you can't sleep, but not due to steroids this time! Plan a party, or a dinner or something to celebrate, you deserve it!

Get someone to teach you how to powder your eyebrows, that's the worst part. Your brows and lashes gradually disappear weeks after chemo is finished! But they grow back superfast, you might look like an unsexy Bruce Willis but use makeup and spray tan. Yes, you tan your head! You'll soon look as well as you'll hopefully feel!

Once you're all done, and you walk out of the chemo unit for the last time, with hugs, laughs and maybe a friend or six, you'll then gradually feel the chemo exiting your body and you'll feel less foggy, less puffy, your jawline and cheek bones will return, even if you didn't notice them disappearing. Your period might come back, hallelujah! People get used to your routine, they become invested and want to celebrate with you, and they want to know how you are. If your people are positive, they make you positive and vice versa. They've been through a big thing watching you too – celebrate with them.

You'll go to the gym and feel just generally unfit compared to the chemo unfit. Your hair will resemble a baby bird, but it will grow back and you'll just be so bloody happy that this chapter is done. Little things won't bother you. You may take risks that you didn't previously. You might not even recognise yourself from pre-BC days. You will start to feel attractive again, and people will say they admire you. You might want to just get on with life, but the truth is, you've just done something huge. You might still have radiotherapy, you might still have endocrine therapy, or surgery, or concerns about your fertility – but this huge chapter is ticked off your list.

Friends will step up, you'll discover new best friends. Some will call you just to see how you're going. Some won't know what the right thing to say is, but they'll be there for you and that's all you need. You might be so bloody over the whole cancer thing, you might be sick of talking about it. You might've been so enthusiastic to help others whilst you were in treatment, but now that it's over you might just want to have a break. But then.... two of your colleagues will be diagnosed, they'll come to you to talk, for advice, to share their experience and you will find the strength and the motivation to pay it forward, to help your friends, to be more than just the young woman who had cancer.

You will get through this, there will be tough days but you're tougher.

Much love,

♡ *Chels*

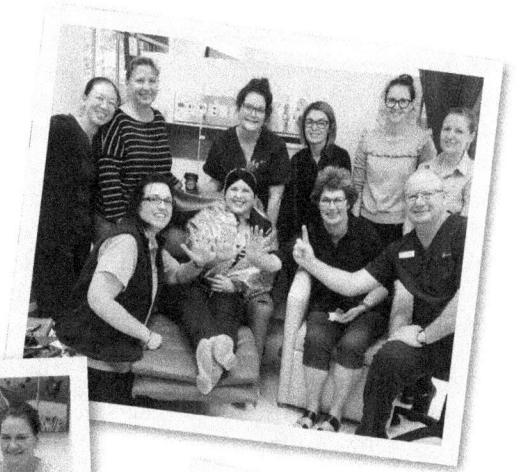

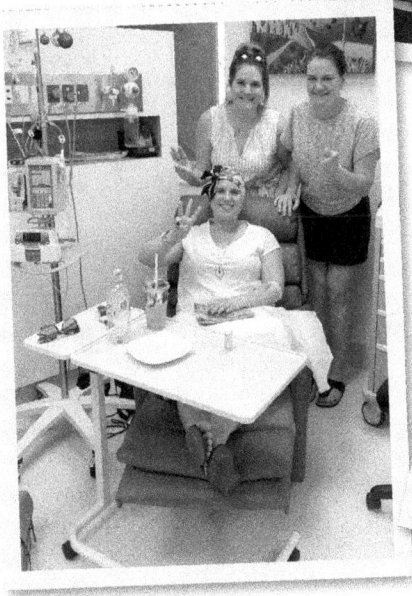

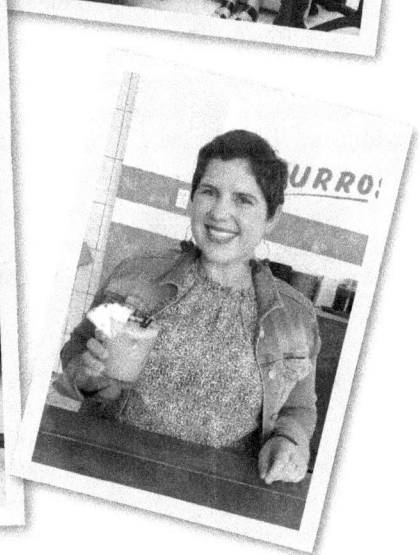

MELLISSA

Dear friend,

I am so sorry. I'm sorry you have to go through this. It is unfair. It doesn't make sense. It shouldn't happen. It shouldn't have happened to me. It shouldn't be happening to you.

I still vividly remember the day I was diagnosed. Seeing the image appear on the screen and, being a doctor, recognising the familiar pattern of calcifications and knowing that it was cancer. Sitting in the waiting room I felt numb, not numb enough though to not feel the pain of the multiple biopsies before being sent home to wait for the results. I remember trying to prepare my mum and my husband for the results. Their optimism that the results would be fine, when I already knew they would not, but holding on to the hope that I might be wrong. Then there was the whirlwind of appointments, and discussions and decisions that followed that no one should have to make, let alone at the age of 37. Our home life was thrown into complete disarray and my toddler girls behaviour deteriorated in response, adding to our already mounting stress.

Life won't ever be the same after a cancer diagnosis. But you'll find a new normal. I've spent a lot of time following my diagnosis and treatment reflecting on meaning and purpose in my return to everyday ordinary life. After a cancer diagnosis, the ordinary things in life, the things we take for granted – like raising a family, going to work, relationships – whilst bringing renewed joy and gratitude, also present additional challenges due to the overlay of fear, grief, loss, trauma, lack of confidence, pain, fatigue, underlying physical, emotional and psychological issues, loss of function and disability. Invisible to the outside world, these can weigh you down and sometimes make what was previously easy and automatic, seem like Mt Everest. My advice to you – don't try to do it alone.

Many people will ask if they can help. Make sure you say yes when they do. Open yourself to receiving help from others and ask for their help when you need it. You may need to direct them in how to best help you in the way you need, whether its drive you to an appointment, help with meals, pick up the kids or a shoulder to cry on.

Be kind to yourself and take time for yourself. It's ok to focus on you. As women and mothers, we are so used to giving much of ourselves to others, putting ourselves last – now is when you need to put your needs first. You will worry about how everyone else will cope, how this will affect those you love, who will pick up the things you normally do. How can the world still turn when life is turned upside down? But you will put one foot in front of the other and find a way to step your way through this challenge. You are strong and resilient and brave. Stronger, more resilient and braver than you think, and you will learn this about yourself. Your journey will be your own journey, but you can take comfort in the company of others who've travelled their own journeys. There can be incredible comfort in connecting with others with similar experiences. Nobody quite understands what you are going through like another person who has been through it. Create a support system around you. Keep the people that matter close to you and spend your time and energy on those who fill your cup.

Be your own patient advocate, don't be afraid to ask for things to be explained so you can understand and make informed decisions, don't let others dismiss your fears or concerns and speak up if needed to ensure you get the care you need.

Wishing you well.

♡ Mellissa

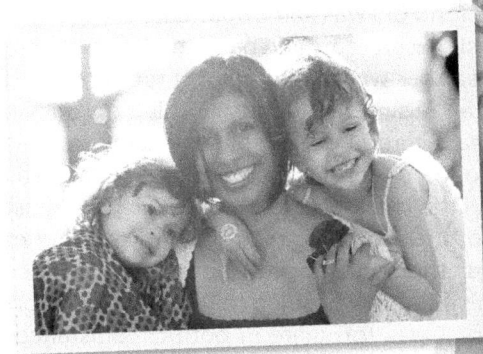

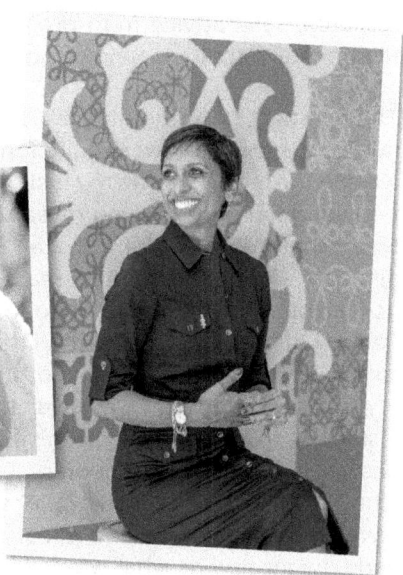

MARG

Hi sweetie,

It's often hard to find the words to say when someone gets a diagnosis of cancer. It's even harder if their diagnosis brings the uncertainty of a future that they had anticipated with family, friends and a career. For many people these days, there is life after cancer but what does that mean? As young women (I was 39 at first diagnosis and 46 at my second – yeah, young!) we go about a busy lives not giving too much consideration to such interruptions but when it hits, it's like a freight train running through your whole body when you hear those words, "sorry, you have cancer". There doesn't seem to be any recollection of what's said after that for many cancer patients. Whilst the doctor is still rambling on about what's next, for most of us those words are still spiralling around our heads with the dreaded thought, will I beat this?

I don't know that the words "I'm sorry you've got cancer" are what you want to hear at this point. I know I hated those words. Why are you sorry? Someone has to get it. Oh God, that someone is me. The world doesn't stop spinning in those first minutes, hours, days and weeks. Your head is full of wonder and not in the best sense of the word. But I ask you to heed this advice, it was my mantra to myself. This wise self-wisdom came into play – I can't change this, so tell me how I roll with the punches? Do your research, seek advice from professionals, prepare yourself mentally for the unknown that is bound to occur.

The prospect of losing my ample sized breasts (that mind you, both my husband and myself were quite fond of) was somewhat daunting. I recall waking the morning after my first mastectomy and bandaged up like what felt like a mummy, bracing myself for what I may think. I recall heading to the bathroom at the hospital, raising my nightie and letting out an almighty sigh. My fabulous breast care nurse by my side said that was not uncommon and others let out a cry or a scream. At that stage, I still had my other breast, so I felt a little lopsided. How was I going to adjust to this? Would any sort of reconstruction help me regain this feeling of my lost womanhood? I was given this soft, temporary prosthesis to place inside my crop top. What? Is this what it was going to feel like? The short answer is NO. It was temporary. I was fortunate in both circumstances (the first diagnosis exensive DCIS and the second a small tumour) not to have to endure chemo and radiation, however radical surgery after very early diagnosis was what was in my favour.

I went on to have a breast reduction of the remaining breast and a recon on the side which was removed. It takes some time, well a fair bit of time, for any sensation to come back. I'm not going to lie, it's limited. I had almost five years of my 'new me' and then an unrelated cancer (this is actually a good thing!) was found in my other breast. This also required removal of my whole breast to decrease my risk. It was a very small but aggressive tumour. This time I couldn't have the expander and straight exchange to a permanent prosthetic breast. I had a lat dorsi reconstruction, taking the muscle from my back to fill the cavity in my chest wall. I then had a small expander in to stretch my skin and then a small implant. Do my breasts look normal? Define normal! They are a permanent part of me and have allowed me to regain my feeling of femininity and womanhood. I have the love and support of an amazing family, this has seen me through the difficult times, and there has been some! It's not all smooth sailing but I believe if you surround yourself with people who love you unconditionally, are prepared to take you on the good and the bad days, and give it all you've got by treating yourself to good physical and mental health, then you have a shot at living your best life.

I have just celebrated my 52nd Birthday. I've celebrated them all in style in the last few years. Old age is a privilege denied to so many...

Take good care,

♡ Marg

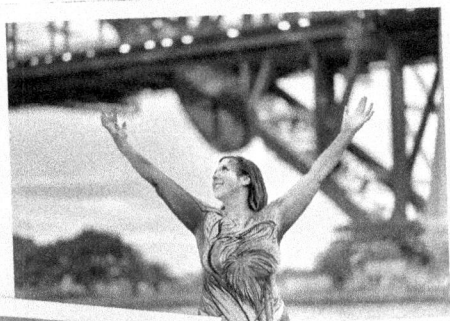

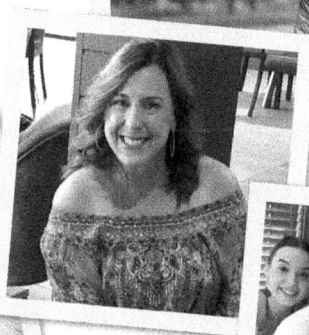

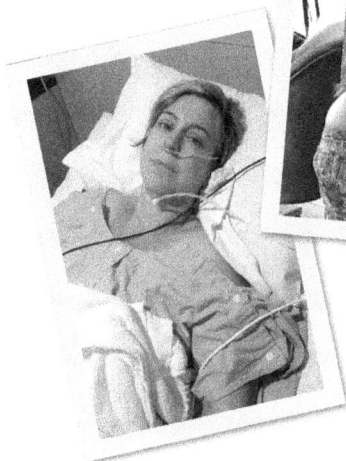

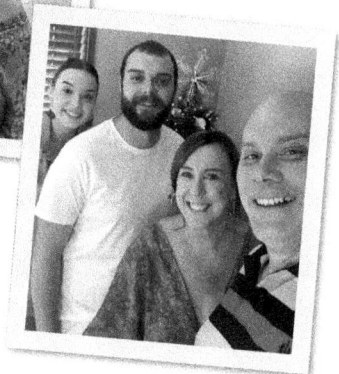

ROBYN

From one warrior to another,

I never thought I would be writing you this letter, but I guess you never expected to be reading it either, huh? Where to start? Well I guess the first thing I want to say to you is, I am sorry. I am so sorry that this is happening to you and that life as you know it has been turned upside down. I'm not going to say something clichéd like 'everything happens for a reason' because three years on and the reasons still escape me. That said, it's important to me that you know, three years on I am happy. Truly happy. I know that right now in this moment you may not be able to see that you will feel happy or joyful again. It may feel like laughter will never again just pass your lips freely as it once did, and your smiles will never come without effort, but they will. You will laugh again, you will smile and you may possibly even make some wildly inappropriate cancer jokes in time, heck knows I do. Light will find a way to creep back in.

One thing I learnt when I joined the club no one wants to be a part of, is we are all pretty funny people. Whether we started out like that, or cancer made us see the importance of finding joy, I don't know, but I do know that some of the most amazing women I have ever had the privilege to meet have walked this path. So while I am deeply sorry you got dealt this hand, know you joined a club filled with incredible people.

As I pondered how best to impart all my cancer kid wisdoms on you, I decided that in sharing my story with you, my advice would be naturally weaved throughout and feel more like the conversation I want to have with you, rather than a checklist. Trust me you will already receive plenty of those!

I celebrated my 30th birthday in October 2015, jetting off with friends to Day Dream Island... I was a new mum to a beautiful little girl, I had a wonderful partner and my whole life was mapped out. I was literally living my best life.

Fast forward to December 2015, I found a lump in my left breast. I didn't pay it much attention but after some motherly prompting I went along to my GP. I went there knowing it was nothing because I was 30, healthy and breast feeding my then five month old, so of course it was nothing. I don't smoke and hardly drink alcohol and had no family history. So to me it was obvious, it had to be mastitis or a cyst, because after all, young women don't get breast cancer, right? So there I was attending the GP and having an ultrasound knowing it was nothing... until it wasn't.

December 22nd 2015, I returned to my GP for my results. I had asked my husband who happened to have the day off to come with me, which still strikes me as one of those weird moments because I would never normally have asked him. I still wonder if on some level I knew something wasn't ok. It was on that day my world stood still. My GP told me I had breast cancer. I vividly remember asking him if I was going to die and he replied, "I don't know". These words still haunt me today, and writing this three years on has had a surprising effect on me. These are not the words you expect to hear at 30. Having cancer at any age is terrible, but to be diagnosed at 30 with a tiny baby and your whole life ahead of you was quite simply devastating, not only for me but for my whole family.

The next few days, I lurched from appointment to appointment, test to test. My stomach dropping with every phone call. I moved between feeling numb and gut wrenching sobs and praying. Making decisions about whether to have IVF or not, do I need a chemo port or would my veins hold up? Mainly wondering when I was going to wake from this nightmare. I would lay awake at night googling everything to do with breast cancer (FYI, Google is not a great way to calm any fear, one minute I had breast cancer and next minute, courtesy of Google, I had cancer and various other rare diseases). My advice a you at this point is take your phone with you to appointments and hit record, that way you can listen to what the doctors are saying when the fog finally lifts on your brain. Take someone you trust with you, armed with the questions that need answering and don't rely on your memory for this, because trust me, your memory will fail you when faced with an event of this magnitude. It will also continue to fail you throughout treatment, because chemo brain is a real thing!

I met my surgeon the day after I was diagnosed and she was a blessing. I dare say, this straight-talking, quick-witted lady may not be everyone's cup of tea, but she immediately instilled confidence in me. She told me what was going to happen, how it would happened and imparted words that still echo for me today – "my girl do not let this mess extinguish your light". Amanda had me prepped and ready for surgery on the 27th of December, telling me she had nothing better planned for Christmas so 'let's get this done'. I asked only one thing of my family that Christmas, no one was to mention the word cancer. I wanted just one more day of normal. Don't be afraid to tell people you love that you want cancer-free zones, conversations and weekends. Cancer has a way of engulfing your whole world in seconds and sometimes you just need it gone. I found very quickly I relished in what my friends and family viewed as 'mundane' conversations. They began to avoid telling me about their 'trivial' problems thinking I was somehow comparing my trials to theirs, or believing I may think less of them for confiding in me. Over the next few months I would lose count of how many times I told my friends 'please tell me about the break up' or 'whinge to me about how your husband doesn't pack the dishwasher'. Yes, this is happening to you, but try not to let this become you. I assure you, even without meeting you, I know you are so much more than this disease.

The day of surgery arrived quickly and my world as it was known to me shifted. My mum moved into my house to care for my daughter, and me, I guess, but that part didn't become obvious until I was home. I am not sure what I had expected, but given I have always been fiercely independent, I couldn't comprehend what it would be like. So I said my goodbyes to my mum and daughter, it would be the first time I'd be away from her, and headed off to hospital to have my breast removed.

When I started to write this, I told myself I would not sugar-coat the story, so in light of this commitment, simply put, this surgery is unkind. It hurts physically and emotionally. I was in a great deal of pain. When I went home it was with drainage bags in both sides and I had nurses check them daily. I cried a lot over the next few days. I would sit in the bath and sob, nothing I can tell you now will adequately prepare you for this, and for that I am sorry. All I can do is give you the practical tips. Make sure you have button up or zip up shirts to wear and know you will need help to sit up, to shower and to dress. But there's no quick tips for the emotional and mental toll this will take, no life hack I can provide. We all just work through this in our own way, on our own terms. So give yourself the space and patience to do it. I left the hospital too quickly, this was my choice. I could have and should have stayed another night or two, but I was too stubborn or foolish or both. I was under some strange delusion that simply by being in my home it would make this situation better, it would hurt less, but it didn't. My advice to you, don't rush home. While home is safe and comforting, recovery is hard. Give yourself a few days, because rushing home will not suddenly make the recovery quicker. In my case, it just made the reality all the more stark. That said, within a week the tubes were out and I attended my sister's wedding ten days later. Now I wouldn't recommend filling your social calendar post-surgery but it was one I couldn't get out of.

I cannot stress enough how important it is to do the physio and exercises they give you once you get clearance, they hurt and it's hard, but it's worth it! As a fit, active person, I never imagined lifting my arm above my head would be hard work and for weeks it was. I slowly regained movement and persevering meant I regained full mobility within a matter of weeks.

It was about the same time, my surgeon Amanda called me with the results of my CT and bone scans. Much like the day of diagnosis, I still remember this call like it was yesterday. I was driving and pulled over to take the call. When I heard her voice I am pretty sure I stopped breathing. I knew why she was calling, her voice boomed down the line "Hello darling it's Amanda... tests are all clear, we got it all, now I must go, I have sick people to speak to". I knew what she was doing, she was aiming for levity, lightness, in a phone call that otherwise would have felt suffocating. For me, she nailed it. I pulled the car over and cried. Relief, joy, happiness. See, I told you that light would find a way to creep in amongst the darkness.

When asked to describe what being diagnosed feels like, I often ask people, have you ever been to the beach and a huge wave comes along and dumps you? You know the feeling when it pulls you to the bottom and the water pressure holds you there? For a few seconds, you genuinely believe you cannot breathe and won't be able to get back to the top, that's cancer. Then the wave subsides and you stand up and breathe. That's what happens when you get your treatment plan. You can breathe again, it gives you purpose, a plan, a way forward. As human beings, we all need direction to orientate ourselves. Make sure you trust your medical team and they will orient you. Don't ever be afraid to get a second opinion or search for a doctor or oncologist who you feel safe with.

Soon after in January of 2016, I started a harsh regime of dose dense chemo for the next eight weeks. Before starting chemo I had to have an injection in my stomach; Zoladex, aka Goserelin or Ryan Gosling to the nurses and me, who struggled to pronounce its shelf name. This is to protect my ovaries from the chemo if I am to have any chance at babies in the future. I still have this each month as part of my treatment as it keeps me in menopause. It's a huge needle and in the early days all of my nurses would play rock/paper/scissors to decide who would administer it. I think it still hurts them more than me if I am being honest. Fingers crossed, it's done its job, but we won't know for another few years until I finish hormone therapy and try for those babies. You see that? Future plans! Do yourself a favour and keep making them. Make them big and bold and vibrant and keep your eyes fixed on them.

The first few rounds of chemo were particularly brutal. My hair fell out almost exactly 14 days from my first treatment. What the doctors forget to tell you is that losing your hair hurts, but to be fair to them, they probably have no idea. My head and scalp hurt until I decided to shave my head at which point, I was bald but no more sore scalp. For me shaving my head was an act of control, it was me showing cancer I was still able to make some choices and call some shots in this misfortune. My friends came over, we had wine and my husband shaved his head and mine. There were tears and laughter, it was easily the worst party I have ever attended but I felt incredibly loved.

Something that has stuck with me throughout this whole experience, even today, is the sense of love and support I was surrounded by. Cancer truly sucks, but people well people are amazing. Plus, it turned out my mum had done a stellar job when I was a baby and must have rotated me well, so no flat spots for me! Some people even said I had a good head for bald! To quote one dear friend who was with me while I shaved my head, "you're not even ugly, you're doing cancer really well". Doctors will also fail to mention you will lose your nose hair. Now this is a real pain because your nose just runs all the time. Sure it's not life threatening but if you want to avoid wiping your nose on your sleeve, carry tissues! My eyebrows went too and so did my lashes, but thankfully you can draw on eyebrows. I recommend this to avoid looking strange, if you have ever seen someone without eyebrows you will know what I mean. You may be thinking, well at least with all this hair loss, I won't have to shave my legs? Well not so fast, the treatment gods somehow weaved their magic and for me at least, my leg hair stayed put! Other advice I received from survivors and the oncology nurses was to gargle salt water to avoid mouth ulcers and keep my nails painted to stop them going yellow through treatment. I am unsure of the validity of this, but I gargled and kept my nails painted and for the most part this worked for me. Regardless, it's a great excuse to get your nails done and sometimes it's the little things that help make us feel brighter when we feel like life has really worn us down.

For me, the worst of chemo came in the first 2-3 days. I generally went for a run before I had treatment, because I knew over the next few days I would only be moving between bed and the couch. I describe the after effect as similar to a hangover on steroids. After my initial dose I was incredibly ill and literally lay in bed for three days with a migraine and nausea, however this was the worst of it and from that point, it really was more like an intense hangover. My advice, if you don't already have it, invest in Netflix or Stan, and no I am not getting any kind of kick back from either streaming service, but days are long when you are literally sitting about and when you wake in the middle of the night, binge watching some new TV show is a far better option than turning to Dr Google. I remember watching TV late at night and feeling sadness about this reality washing over me, still not really believing this was my life, and then letting the tears flow. Someone very smart told me, 'don't cry to quit, cry to keep going; you're already in pain, you might as well get rewarded for it'.

During those first few days post chemo I'd feel ill, but hungry, thanks to the steroids they give you to minimise nausea. 'Get cancer they said, you'll lose weight they said'.... well no one actually ever said that to me, but you know, everyone thinks it! That's because no one knows about the steroids!

So let me take a minute to fill you in on Dexamethasone, or Dex, as it's affectionately known. Well not to me because I have no fondness for this medication at ALL. In fairness, 'Dex' is pretty good at keeping the nausea at bay and the hunger up. It's also not bad at keeping you awake, and for me at least, turning me into the hulk at times. To make up for this I would give my nearest and dearest a blanket apology on chemo day to cover me for what was bound to be a wild ride for us all over the next 72 hours. My go to food post chemo included Smith's plain chips, lemonade icy poles and cheeseburgers! To give you an idea of what I was like in those first few days, I remember crying once because no one would go and get me a cheeseburger. Sure, I admit they are delicious, but prior to getting sick I can hand on heart say, McDonalds was not really something I ate. Yet here I was crying over the absence of a cheeseburger! I messaged my dad and had a full blown toddler fit about it... and as all good Dad's do, he came bearing cheeseburgers. I maintain this reaction was purely a result of the medication!

Once those first few days passed I made sure to get out and go for a walk and get fresh air. The one thing I found that truly helped with fatigue was walking. Even those times where I was so flat I couldn't imagine moving, I would head out for a cruise around the block and this made a huge difference. If you can keep active, do so. Some days it may feel hard or even impossible but it makes for a smoother recovery and better mental health. Other important things to remember, if you find yourself on 'top shelf' chemo (the red stuff), you will pee red after treatment. Don't panic, it's not blood, just chemicals. Feel better? You will have to double flush the toilet (ideally if you have two toilets, keep one for yourself) and if by the chance the mood strikes you to get intimate – wear protection, him not you! Your vagina will literally be a little radioactive gem and may send him to the emergency department with an intense burning... (or so I have heard).

During dose dense chemo I also needed to self-inject after each dose for the first few days to allow my white cells to bounce back for the next round. Despite everything else happening to me, I just couldn't bring myself to do this and my husband took it on for me. A small act that meant so much. Don't feel bad, you are not a burden, simply outsource what you cannot manage. These injections meant my bones ached at night but to be fair, between the nausea, muscle aches and insane hot flushes, what's a little bone ache between friends? Panadol works a treat in these times, and I found having it at night before bed meant that with any luck, I would snooze through the aching.

Now, before I move on, I need to tell you why I am making sure to cover off on all the side effects that happened to me. It's definitely not to scare you because, quite frankly, it doesn't actually get more scary than being diagnosed with cancer. It's to make sure you know what may happen. I found that with treatment, knowledge is power and that is pretty important when you feel powerless. Having this knowledge also stopped me from freaking out at every ache or pain (because trust me, that too is going to happen). Knowing that what I was feeling and what was happening to my body was common helped me to manage that stress... a little bit anyway.

After eight weeks of this wonderful cocktail blend, I moved onto Paclitaxel. I can't believe I am actually writing this, but I didn't really mind it. It was a weekly appointment that didn't take as long as the initial regime and didn't leave me feeling sick. I still struggled to sleep so I would find myself working out or cleaning at 3am, but man did my house get clean. However, not everything in the Taxol camp was roses. By about week three I developed a horrible rash all over my face, almost like I was burnt. Once again they filled me to the brim with steroids which seemed to be effective. I had a few blood noses and was lucky enough to develop constipation and haemorrhoids to boot. Who said this chemo lark isn't just a big old bag of fun? There truly is no limit to the joys of treatment! The upshot, my hair started to grow back and I had not one blemish on my skin! It was around this time I felt like I could see a light at the end of the tunnel.

It was also about this time in my journey that I learnt, for me at least, cancer was a war, not just a battle. A marathon, not a sprint. Sometimes cancer would have little victories and I'd feel sad, scared or angry but I soon got really good at reminding myself I too had victories. Successfully completing chemo, recovering post-surgery and taking back my life, pulling myself out of this hell inch by inch. I knew the big wins were going to be mine and eventually I would win the war. My advice, if you are blessed enough to have wonderful friends, family and people in your world, make sure they help remind you all of the ways you are kicking its ass. Sometimes amongst the side effects, fatigue and the enormity of what we have gone through, and what still lies ahead, it's easy to forget the wins. My friends and I also made sure to find ways to smile. By this time we had all gotten pretty sick of hearing the word 'journey'. Trust me, you may also feel this way by the time you finish treatment or heck before you even start! I swear every person you meet will use this term. So my friends and I decided to start finding and using alternatives from a thesaurus; it was our little game. I'm not going to lie, people did shoot me some puzzled looks when I would talk about my voyage or odyssey, but once again through our laughter, those bits of light I mentioned just kept creeping on in.

By this point you will also have also been inundated by well-meaning friends and loved ones... Without a doubt, you will receive more candles and different varieties of tea than you ever knew existed! Hopefully someone had the good sense to show you this letter! Some people may keep their distance and that's tough to accept. I guess it's because it's hard for people to know what to say, and sometimes when we are faced with our own mortality it's simply too scary. Then there are other people you will wish would stay away! They will send you links and tag you in every cancer cure known to man, from some rare fruit found only in a remote village in Nepal, to eating your body weight in pineapple enzymes. I have heard and seen them all and soon so will you.

I still remember seeing a well-meaning and lovely work colleague, she hugged me tight and made sure I knew I was loved after being diagnosed, right before telling me with tears in her eyes "you're not going to die like my friend". My response to this? "I bloody hope not". When I think back on this now I laugh, because I have learnt to be forgiving of people as they stumble to find the right words. My advice for dealing with well-meaning people? Channel your inner Elsa and 'let it go, let it go, let it go'. Until I was diagnosed, I also didn't know what to say to someone with cancer, so remember most people are good, they care and love you. However, remembering how to be patient and gracious with people suffering foot in mouth can be a challenge when you are shot full of drugs and scrambling to make sense of what is happening to you! I found for me, taking this forgiving approach kept me in a better frame of mind and that's what's important. Stewing on the awkward and inappropriate comments that you are bound to hear over the next 12 months will only add to your load, not lighten it.

You will hear every second person tell you to be positive. My advice here is twofold. Again, channel your inner Elsa, but also for what it's worth, much like that rare fruit in Nepal, positivity won't cure cancer, but trust me, it makes you a whole lot more bearable to be around. Now that doesn't mean that I am advocating for fake positivity, but being the president and chairman of your own pity party also won't improve your prognosis. There are some things that I found comforting when I found myself surrounded by fear. I found faith, sometimes all out blind faith is a true blessing. I would religiously read survivors statistics for Australia, because they are pretty darn good, and our scientists are some of the best in the world! So when you feel yourself falling into that hole, where bone-deep, blood-chilling fear hides, think of those scientists, think of those stats and remember, while positivity won't cure cancer, it certainly isn't going to hamper recovery.

While I am laying it all out, there are other things not related to medication or surgery or diagnosis that are taxing. For me, managing other people's emotions felt like a full-time job sometimes. I remember trying not to fall apart in front of my husband in the early days because I wanted to be strong and brave for him. Little did I know, he was doing the same thing. It turns out, when we actually got brave and talked it out, he was able to tell me he'd been crying each day on his way to work so I wouldn't see. That was a like a punch in the guts. Having cancer sucks, but watching someone you love have cancer sucks on a whole different level. A completely hopeless level, so be kind to those who love you. Cancer isn't just affecting you, it affects everyone who you love and loves you. Sure we got dealt the truly shitty card, but watching someone you love hurt is no walk in the park either.

Going through treatment and having a young baby at home was emotionally gruelling and heartbreaking for me. Firstly, having to wean her from me in a matter of days and feel like that bond was being ripped away was devastating. Still today I chalk that up to one of the harder moments in this whole mess, which says something, because to date I have had six months of chemo, 12 months of Herceptin, six weeks of radiation and four surgeries! Never underestimate the emotional impact of this experience. It's the emotional scars that I found, extend far deeper and last far longer than the physical ones. I could see the impact my treatment had on my daughter, having so many people in and out of our home, assisting me to care for her took a toll on her emotions at times too. In these moments I found myself more sensitive and resentful about not being able to care for my daughter the way other mums could. Although I was grateful and appreciated the support and love of friends and family, gratitude isn't always so easy in times like this. My advice you ask? If you can find jobs for people to do, then do it. It makes them feel better and useful, even if it's busy work. If you need or want something done in a particular way, just tell them. It will save a hell of a lot of tears and anger when the towels are folded incorrectly and you find yourself a screaming crying mess... because that happens too; incredible emotional reactions to seemingly small things. My theory is, that for me at least, I spent a lot of time saying how fine I was, that sometimes all my fears and sadness spilled out about things that I felt were tangible. It felt easier and more acceptable to get upset about these things, than to try to express the sadness and heartbreak I felt about not being able to hold my baby when she cried because I'd just had chemotherapy, or how unfair I felt this situation was. Be kind to yourself. You don't have to be a warrior every day, sometimes you just need to let the tears come and not explain them away or even find a reason for them. My experience of cancer and treatment is that it gets harder before it gets easier. It will get better but you just have to get through that hard stuff first, and there ain't no short cut. So surround yourself with amazing people who will pick you up when you hit rock bottom, or that will sit with you there for a little, but that won't let you move there indefinitely.

The day I finished chemo the oncology nurses spoilt me with balloons and coffee and treats. My friends came to celebrate with me over pizza and overall I felt pure joy. It's hard to believe that you can feel so happy during such dark times, but I did. Once again, that light I mentioned earlier finding ways to slip back into my life.

And then there was radiation. During the initial appointment they will spend what feels like hours measuring and getting precise tiny tattoo dots on your skin which will ensure accurate treatment. Be prepared to lay very, very still and be very, very bored. They will try to be respectful about laying on the table with your chest exposed but by this stage, I had lost count of how many people had seen me topless, so while it was very kind, I found it a little bizarre. They covered my flat chest in a second skin like plastic which was to protect me from burning. Sadly it did not take well to my skin, something I have heard is common in young women as our skin is quite 'elasticy' thanks to our young age! In any sense, it came off by the second week and with four weeks to go, I burned like a crisp! I had some great cream that I bought online called Aquaphor. It really helped soothe and repair my skin. Radiation for me had a cumulative impact. I grew more and more tired as the weeks went on. It didn't help that I travelled just over 100km each way for my 8 minute treatment. Make sure you have a good playlist if you need to travel for any appointments. For me personally, I hated radiation more than chemo, which shocks a bunch of people, usually doctors!

So let me think, I've covered off on chemo, radiation and mastectomies amongst the other highlights. Who said cancer wasn't glam? Fast forward 12 months and I was finally allowed to have my reconstruction. I had to wait 12 months to allow my body to heal from radiation. Worth noting was that my oncological surgeon left as much excess skin as she could to allow the plastic surgeon something to work with. So if you are thinking you would like reconstruction then talk to the surgeon about this. It doesn't look as neat in the initial stages but certainly makes a world of difference to the final product. I was unable to have my implants done during my initial mastectomy because I was having radiation and this is not recommended as it damages the implant and can cause a whole bunch of issues. I had to have expanders initially before my definitive implants as radiation had caused significant damage to my skin, making it very tight. This meant I would see the doctor every few weeks at the clinic where he would fill the expander each time with saline increasing the volume bit by bit. Some people have described this as painful, but this was not my experience. It felt like pressure and it was a bit uncomfortable or tight for the next day or so but nothing that caused me pain or even caused me to reach for Panadol. While some people I have spoken to struggled with expanders, I found them to be ok. The idea behind the expanders is to stretch the skin to allow the final implant to look better. I have seen reconstruction done with and without expanders and am personally glad my plastic surgeon went this way. It meant additional surgery but gave me a better overall appearance. This is a very personal choice, as is the decision to have reconstruction at all. Take your time in deciding this, make sure to speak with people and hell, ask to see their boobs if given the opportunity! It's the only way to be sure and fully understand what you may end up with.

I was recently presented with another perplexing question; to nipple or not to nipple? Again not really something I had imagined having to consider, and after a lot of deliberation, debate and viewing of breasts,

I made the decision to have 3D nipple tattooing, and I am pleased I did.

I decided throughout treatment I would not let it get the better of me physically and as someone who already ran prior to getting diagnosed, I put focus and energy on doing this again. My goal was to compete in a half marathon following treatment, which I did in January 2017, literally 12 months after I started chemotherapy. Then I did a few more. What I found was this built my confidence and made me feel in control. Don't worry I'm not about to tell you to start running marathons, but I am going to encourage you to find something you enjoy, something that connects you with the you, that you were before the C word came intruding into your life, and if you can, invest energy into this.

I still check in with my surgeon and oncologist once a year. It's weird because after being thrown head first into appointments and treatments, you are suddenly and abruptly let go. Despite how I thought I would feel when treatment finished, I actually found myself scared and that was when I struggled the most mentally. I thought I would be elated and on top of the world, yet I feared what would happen without chemo? Somewhere along the line, chemo and treatment had become a safety net and as quickly as it sucked me in, it spat me back out, and I was left fending for myself again. Well not completely, but that's how it felt. Having something to put my energy and focus into that was about me as a person and not cancer, helped me work through that fear and tethered me to something when I needed it most. It's also the hardest time, because your hair has grown back and you don't have weekly appointments anymore so in everyone's eyes you're better now, right?

I am well into my hormone therapy, 3 years to be precise. It's a tablet each day and a monthly injection. I am looking at another two years on the Zoladex and Examastane combo, so what does that look like in reality? Bone and joint aches, hot flushes and fatigue (which to be fair is probably a combination of the drugs, the hot flushes that mean I toss and turn at night and being a mum) and another drug to stop my bones from developing osteoporosis. This June, it will be three years post treatment. I'm not going to lie to you and be all Mary Sunshine over here. It has not been without stress and fear, that all of us in this club learn to live with. I'm learning to calm my head and reassure myself that every ache and pain I feel isn't cancer coming back. Sometimes I let the fact that I feel like a 65 year old in a 33 year old's body get me down but for the most part I choose gratitude. I choose gratitude and joy, and choose not to focus on the days I am flat and exhausted. Some cancer survivors I know call this their 'new normal'. I really hate that term, but for now it's all we've got until, of course, my friends and I can thesaurus it and find a whole new lingo for us to start using.

Throughout diagnosis, treatment and recovery I found connecting with someone who had walked this path before me, was invaluable. So I made sure that when I finished my treatment to take time for those women like me that were still to come. That's why I am writing this now.

Shortly after I finished treatment, a friend of mine received the shocking blow that she too had breast cancer. In October of 2018 she wrote something to describe my support of herself, other young women and cancer research – "She looks toward the future and advocates hard to change the historical course of breast cancer. But importantly, she also looks back. Not to complain or dwell. She walks back into the storm to grab the hand of the next young woman diagnosed...". Her words reminded me why it's important to keep raising awareness and keep sharing our stories; it reminds us we are not alone. I hope this letter finds you, obviously not well, or you wouldn't be reading it. But this is me grabbing your hand, walking beside you and offering you hope, shining my light into your darkness, until yours has the strength to shine bright once again.

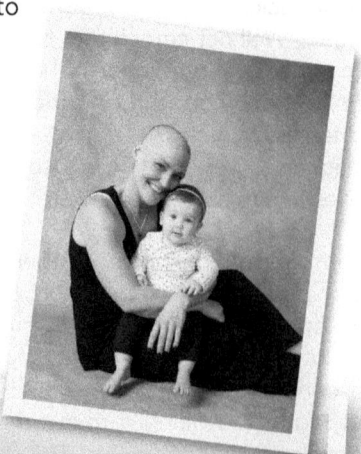

From one warrior to another.

♡ *Robyn*

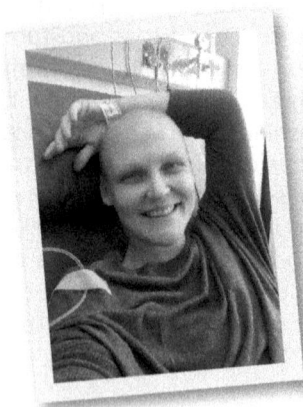

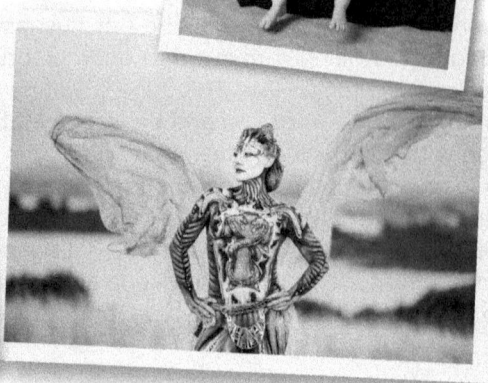

ACKNOWLEDGEMENTS

Where would we be in life without the people who support us? Breast cancer is many things and one of the most important things it taught me was to be thankful for the things that I didn't even know were my privilege. Health, and especially good health, is never something we should take for granted. I speak on behalf of all breast cancer patients when I say we are so grateful for the people in our lives who have supported us through these traumatic journeys. For all of the people who held our hands, helped us with our homes and our families, shared the good and awful times, and have been there through it all, you are the silver lining in this terrible storm.

We live in an age where women are living beyond breast cancer. We live in a country where we can access world-class healthcare. We're able to share our stories because we faced this mountain and did not let it defeat us.

Everything changed that fateful day when I heard the words "you've got breast cancer". My life will never be the same, but I got to meet people, and do and see and feel things that I would never have before.

I want to thank all the beautiful women (Rachel, Claire, Emma, Hayley, Sue, Jess B, Michelle, Belinda, Sam, Tina, Chelsea, Mellissa, Marg, Jess W and Robyn) who have bravely shared their intimate and personal experiences in the hope that we can make a difference for the next woman who hears those difficult words. You're all amazing, beautiful, strong, resilient and extraordinary women!

I also want to thank my very dear friend Sharon who pulled this book together and believes so dearly in what our mission is trying to achieve. When I talk about the people who I would never have met, I'm so grateful for you.

Lastly to you, thank you for reading this book, whether you've just joined the club that no one wants to join or your supporting somebody who is. We hope our stories will inspire you and reassure you that you are not alone and you too can get through this.

♡ *Rachelle*

Founder, So Brave – Australia's Young Women's Breast Cancer Charity

MY STORY

We'd love you to share your story, and know how cathartic writing can be in dealing with the array of emotions a diagnosis can be. Feel free to share yours here, and maybe one day, share it with a friend who's where you are now.

Take care xx

_____

_____

_____

_____

_____

_____

_____

_____

_____

_____

_____

_____

_____

_____

_____

_____

_____

_____